ONCOLOGY NURSING SOCIETY

Safe Handling of Hazardous Drugs

SECOND EDITION

EDITED BY
MARTHA POLOVICH, PhD, RN, AOCN®

Oncology Nursing Society
Pittsburgh, PA

ONS Publications Department
Interim Publisher and Director of Publications: Barbara Sigler, RN, MNEd
Managing Editor: Lisa M. George, BA
Technical Content Editor: Angela D. Klimaszewski, RN, MSN
Staff Editor: Amy Nicoletti, BA
Copy Editor: Laura Pinchot, BA
Graphic Designer: Dany Sjoen

Copyright © 2011 by the Oncology Nursing Society. All rights reserved. No part of the material protected by this copyright may be reproduced or utilized in any form, electronic or mechanical, including photocopying, recording, or by an information storage and retrieval system, without written permission from the copyright owner. For information, write to the Oncology Nursing Society, 125 Enterprise Drive, Pittsburgh, PA 15275-1214, or visit www.ons.org/publications.

First printing, January 2011
Second printing, January 2012

Library of Congress Cataloging-in-Publication Data

Safe handling of hazardous drugs / edited by Martha Polovich. – 2nd ed.
    p. ; cm.
  Includes bibliographical references and index.
  ISBN 978-1-935864-00-4 (alk. paper)
  1. Drugs–Safety measures. I. Polovich, Martha. II. Oncology Nursing Society.
  [DNLM: 1. Hazardous Substances. 2. Evidence-Based Practice. 3. Occupational Exposure–prevention & control. 4. Pharmaceutical Preparations–adverse effects. WA 487.5.H4]
  RS92.S24 2011
  615'.10289–dc22

                                                                                                 2010040303

Publisher's Note

This book is published by the Oncology Nursing Society (ONS). ONS neither represents nor guarantees that the practices described herein will, if followed, ensure safe and effective patient care. The recommendations contained in this book reflect ONS's judgment regarding the state of general knowledge and practice in the field as of the date of publication. The recommendations may not be appropriate for use in all circumstances. Those who use this book should make their own determinations regarding specific safe and appropriate patient-care practices, taking into account the personnel, equipment, and practices available at the hospital or other facility at which they are located. The editor and publisher cannot be held responsible for any liability incurred as a consequence from the use or application of any of the contents of this book. Figures and tables are used as examples only. They are not meant to be all-inclusive, nor do they represent endorsement of any particular institution by ONS. Mention of specific products and opinions related to those products do not indicate or imply endorsement by ONS. Web sites mentioned are provided for information only; the hosts are responsible for their own content and availability. Unless otherwise indicated, dollar amounts reflect U.S. dollars.

ONS publications are originally published in English. Publishers wishing to translate ONS publications must contact ONS about licensing arrangements. ONS publications cannot be translated without obtaining written permission from ONS. (Individual tables and figures that are reprinted or adapted require additional permission from the original source.) Because translations from English may not always be accurate or precise, ONS disclaims any responsibility for inaccuracies in words or meaning that may occur as a result of the translation. Readers relying on precise information should check the original English version.

Printed in the United States of America

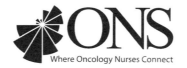

Oncology Nursing Society
Integrity • Innovation • Stewardship • Advocacy • Excellence • Inclusiveness

Contributors

Editor

Martha Polovich, PhD, RN, AOCN®
Associate Director, Clinical Practice
Duke Oncology Network
Durham, North Carolina
Introduction; Evidence for Occupational Hazardous Drug Exposure; Personal Protective Equipment

Authors

Deborah L. Bolton, RN, MN, CNS-FNP, AOCNS®, AOCNP®
Medical Oncology Clinical Nurse Specialist
Marin General Hospital
Greenbrae, California
Nurse Practitioner
Stay Well Research
Northridge, California
Drug Administration

Seth Eisenberg, RN, ADN, OCN®
Professional Practice Coordinator, Infusion
  Services
Seattle Cancer Care Alliance
Seattle, Washington
Drug Administration; Post-Administration Issues; Management of Spills

Eileen M. Glynn-Tucker, RN, MS
Educator and Consultant
Green Oaks, Illinois
Definition of Hazardous Drugs; Adverse Effects of Hazardous Drug Exposure; Linen Handling

Josie Howard-Ruben, MS, RN, APN-CNS, AOCN®
Oncology Clinical Development Specialist/
  Lead Nurse Planner
Advocate Health Care
Park Ridge, Illinois
Staff Education and Training

Melissa A. McDiarmid, MD, MPH, DABT
Professor of Medicine
University of Maryland School of Medicine
Baltimore, Maryland
Medical Surveillance of Healthcare Workers Handling Hazardous Drugs

Luci A. Power, MS, RPh
Senior Consultant
Power Enterprises
San Francisco, California
Hierarchy of Controls; Drug Compounding; Safety Measures

Charlotte A. Smith, RPh, MS
Director, PharmEcology Services
WM Healthcare Solutions, Inc.
Houston, Texas
Disposal of Hazardous Drugs*

Field Reviewers

Carol Stein Blecher, RN, MS, AOCN®, APNC
Advanced Practice Nurse/Clinical Educator
Trinitas Comprehensive Cancer Center
Elizabeth, New Jersey

Kimberly George, MSN, RN, ACNS-BC, OCN®
Clinical Nurse Specialist, Oncology/Hematology
United Regional Health Care System
Wichita Falls, Texas

Kristine B. LeFebvre, MSN, RN, AOCN®
Project Manager, Education
Oncology Nursing Society
Pittsburgh, Pennsylvania

MiKaela M. Olsen, RN, MS, OCN®
Oncology and Bone Marrow Transplant Clinical Nurse Specialist
The Sidney Kimmel Comprehensive Cancer Center at Johns Hopkins Hospital
Baltimore, Maryland

Debra L. Winkeljohn, RN, MSN, AOCN®, CNS
Clinical Director
Hematology Oncology Associates
Albuquerque, New Mexico

* This chapter reflects the personal opinions of the author and does not necessarily represent the views of WM Healthcare Solutions or Waste Management.

Disclosure

Editors and authors of books and guidelines provided by the Oncology Nursing Society are expected to disclose to the readers any significant financial interest or other relationships with the manufacturer(s) of any commercial products.

A vested interest may be considered to exist if a contributor is affiliated with or has a financial interest in commercial organizations that may have a direct or indirect interest in the subject matter. A "financial interest" may include, but is not limited to, being a shareholder in the organization; being an employee of the commercial organization; serving on an organization's speakers bureau; or receiving research from the organization. An "affiliation" may be holding a position on an advisory board or some other role of benefit to the commercial organization. Vested interest statements appear in the front matter for each publication.

Contributors are expected to disclose any unlabeled or investigational use of products discussed in their content. This information is acknowledged solely for the information of the readers.

The contributors provided the following disclosure and vested interest information:

Martha Polovich, PhD, RN, AOCN®: honoraria, ICU Medical
Seth Eisenberg, RN, ADN, OCN®: honoraria, Medical Learning Institute, ProCE
Luci A. Power, MS, RPh: honoraria, ProCE

Contents

Abbreviations Used vii

Clinical Update to Oncology Nursing Society Safe Handling Guidelines
    Regarding Surface Safe® viii

Introduction 1

Definition of Hazardous Drugs 3

Adverse Effects of Hazardous Drug Exposure 4

Evidence for Occupational Hazardous Drug Exposure 11

Hierarchy of Controls 18

Drug Compounding 27

Safety Measures 34

Drug Administration 35

Post-Administration Issues 47

Management of Spills 53

Medical Surveillance of Healthcare Workers Handling Hazardous Drugs 58

Staff Education and Training 66

References 73

Appendix A. Hazardous Drug Administration Safe Handling Checklist 83

Appendix B. Hazardous Drug Administration Practicum for RNs 84

Index 87

Abbreviations Used

ACPH—air changes per hour
AHFS—American Hospital Formulary Services
ASHP—American Society of Health-System Pharmacists
ASTM—American Society for Testing and Materials
BBB—blood-brain barrier
BSC—biologic safety cabinet
CACI—compounding aseptic containment isolator
CETA—Controlled Environment Testing Association
CNS—central nervous system
CSF—cerebrospinal fluid
CSP—compounded sterile preparation
CSTD—closed-system drug transfer device
EPA—U.S. Environmental Protection Agency
HCW—healthcare worker
HD—hazardous drug
HEPA—high-efficiency particulate air
IARC—International Agency for Research on Cancer
IP—intraperitoneal
ISO—International Organization for Standardization
M—mole/molarity
MPE—malignant pleural effusion
MSDS—material safety data sheet
NCI—National Cancer Institute
NIOSH—National Institute for Occupational Safety and Health
ONS—Oncology Nursing Society
OR—operating room
OSHA—Occupational Safety and Health Administration
PEC—primary engineering control
PPE—personal protective equipment
RCRA—Resource Conservation and Recovery Act
USP—U.S. Pharmacopeia

Clinical Update to Oncology Nursing Society Safe Handling Guidelines Regarding Surface Safe®

The second edition of the Oncology Nursing Society (ONS) guidelines *Safe Handling of Hazardous Drugs*, published in February 2011, makes reference to the use of Surface Safe® solution, marketed by Hospira, Inc., for decontaminating primary engineering controls (see pp. 30, 55, and 56 in the publication). Subsequent to the publication of the ONS guidelines, Hospira notified its customers that it will no longer be marketing this product. Currently, no commercially available alternative has been determined. ONS will issue an alert once an appropriate alternative product has been identified.

Much support for the use of chlorine bleach exists in the general decontamination references and in specific drug material safety data sheets from manufacturers. Sodium thiosulfate is a known deactivating agent for a number of chemotherapy drugs and is also a specific neutralizer for chlorine bleach.

To approximate the same concentration as is available in Surface Safe (2% sodium hypochlorite),

- Mix approximately half standard Clorox® (5.25%; Clorox® Ultra is more concentrated) with half sterile water for irrigation (SWFI).
- Add a small amount of liquid detergent (not too much or it will be hard to rinse).

For complete decontamination of a biologic safety cabinet, including under the work tray, about 1 liter of the bleach and detergent mixture is needed. This mixture will accomplish cleaning (detergent), removal of drug residue (towelette with proper disposal), and deactivation of some hazardous drugs and most microbes (bleach). Chlorine bleach at 2% concentration is an excellent disinfectant—better than alcohol—and a sporicide, which alcohol is not.

Because chlorine bleach can damage stainless steel surfaces, follow with sodium thiosulfate solution. The thiosulfate neutralizes the bleach to avoid this damage. The sodium thiosulfate also deactivates some hazardous drugs (e.g., platinum compounds, mechlorethamine). To approximate the same concentration as in Surface Safe (1.0%), mix sodium thiosulfate with SWFI. The thiosulfate may be available in 10% or 25% solution, which requires about 1:10 or 1:25 dilution with SWFI. The neutralization process creates NaCl—salt—which must be rinsed thoroughly with SWFI to remove.

Use gauze pads (4 × 4) for each step of the process, and dispose of them as chemotherapy waste.

1. Bleach/detergent solution
2. Sodium thiosulfate solution
3. SWFI rinse

References

Castegnaro, M., De Meo, M.D., Laget, M., Michelon, J., Garren, L., Sportouch, M.H., & Hansel, S. (1997). Chemical degradation of wastes of antineoplastic agents. 2: Six anthracyclines: Idarubicin, doxorubicin, epirubicin, pirarubicin, aclarubicin and daunorubicin. *International Archives of Occupational and Environmental Health, 70,* 378–384. doi:10.1007/s004200050232

Gonzalez, R., & Massoomi, F.F. (2010). Manufacturers' recommendations for handling spilled hazardous drugs. *American Journal of Health-System Pharmacy, 67,* 1985–1986. doi:10.2146/ajhp100137

Hansel, S., Castegnaro, M., Sportouch, M.H., De Meo, M., Milhavet, J.C., Laget, M., & Dumenil, G. (1997). Chemical degradation of wastes of antineoplastic agents: Cyclophosphamide, ifosfamide and melphalan. *International Archives of Occupational and Environmental Health, 69,* 109–114. doi:10.1007/s004200050124

Hospira, Inc. (n.d.). Surface Safe® packets. Retrieved from http://www.hospira.com/Products/surfacesafe.aspx

Roberts, S., Khammo, N., McDonnell, G., & Sewell, G.J. (2006). Studies on the decontamination of surfaces exposed to cytotoxic drugs in chemotherapy workstations. *Journal of Oncology Pharmacy Practice, 12,* 95–104. doi:10.1177/1078155206070439

Introduction

The issue of healthcare worker (HCW) exposure to hazardous drugs (HDs) first emerged in 1979. Guidelines for the safe handling of HDs have been available for more than 20 years. Although the recommended guidelines have not changed significantly during that time, the information related to the potential for occupational exposure has changed. Evidence of contamination in healthcare work environments with HDs has been reported in the occupational health literature since the early 1990s. This information regarding potential health risks, considered with the fact that nearly six million HCWs handle HDs (U.S. Bureau of Labor Statistics, 2009), emphasizes the need to focus on HD safe handling. Much of the evidence we present from the literature is old, but it still has value. We have *not* solved the problem of occupational HD exposure.

This manual is based on the recommendations of the Oncology Nursing Society (ONS), the Occupational Safety and Health Administration (OSHA), and the American Society of Health-System Pharmacists (ASHP, formerly the American Society of Hospital Pharmacists). Its intent is to help to translate the recommendations into practice for nurses who handle HDs in the care of patients. More importantly, nurses are encouraged to critically examine their work practices in order to identify activities that might result in HD exposure and to change practices that might put themselves and their colleagues at risk.

In preparing the update to these guidelines, the authors searched the PubMed system of the National Library of Medicine using the following key words: *antineoplastic agents, hazardous drugs,* and *occupational exposure.* Articles were limited to those published in the English language in peer-reviewed journals from 2000 forward. Older publications considered classic references are also included.

Further searches of the medical literature were conducted (based on initial findings, group feedback, and authors' experience) to identify additional and relevant materials. In addition to searching peer-reviewed publications, the authors searched Web sites of known domestic or international medical organizations or professional societies involved in producing relevant materials (e.g., reports, white papers, official announcements) related to hazardous drug topics. The authors sought to identify literature that would point to recommended evidence-based standards of practice or specific quality measures that had been developed by healthcare organizations or specialty societies. Web sites of the following organizations were searched:

- www.ons.org
- www.ashp.org
- www.cdc.gov/niosh/
- www.OSHA.gov

Findings derived from these searches were used to generate additional searches for guidelines published in the United States and abroad.

Definition of Hazardous Drugs

HDs require careful handling by healthcare personnel and others who come in contact with them to minimize the adverse health effects of exposure and reduce contamination of the workplace. A definition of HDs is essential so that clinicians recognize the drugs for which the safe handling recommendations apply. Drugs are classified as hazardous when they possess any one of the following six characteristics (ASHP, 1990, 2006; National Institute for Occupational Safety and Health [NIOSH], 2004).

- **Genotoxicity**, or the ability to cause a change or mutation in genetic material; a mutagen.
- **Carcinogenicity**, or the ability to cause cancer in humans, animal models, or both; a carcinogen. The International Agency for Research on Cancer (IARC) classifies agents as carcinogens if they are capable of increasing the incidence of cancers, reducing the latency period before cancer development, or increasing the severity of growth of a malignancy. In some cases, an agent's ability to induce benign tumors was also evidence used to classify an agent as a carcinogen (IARC, 2006).
- **Teratogenicity**, or the ability to cause defects in fetal development or fetal malformation; a teratogen.
- **Fertility impairment or reproductive toxicity.**
- **Serious organ toxicity at low doses** in humans or animal models.
- **Chemical structure and toxicity profile that mimic existing drugs determined to be hazardous** by the five previous criteria. This additional criterion to the definition of HDs was first published by NIOSH in 2004 and serves as a reminder that new drugs should be critically evaluated using existing information and extrapolating data from similar agents. ASHP (2006) recommends that organizations evaluate the hazardous potential for all drugs, approved and investigational, when they are first introduced into the facility.

HDs may include antineoplastic or cytotoxic agents, biologic agents, antiviral agents, immunosuppressive agents, and drugs from other classes. OSHA (1995) recommends that all investigational agents be regarded as potentially hazardous until information establishing their safety becomes available. In the event that data provided to the principal investigator about an investigational agent are insufficient to make a decision, it is prudent to handle the agent as though it is hazardous (ASHP, 2006; NIOSH, 2004). ASHP (2006) specifies that all drugs should be considered hazardous if the information obtained about the drug is insufficient to make an informed decision as to whether it is hazardous. Certainly, healthcare providers must recognize that erring on the side of caution is essential to protecting workers' health and safety and the safety of the work environment.

The first step for organizations in creating an environment that is safe from HD exposure is to determine what HDs are used in the setting. Organizations should develop a list of all HDs used and ensure that a method is in place to regularly review and update the list. A comprehensive list of all drugs currently considered hazardous does not exist in the literature. Given the large number of new drug approvals each year, organizations must have a process for evaluating the medications they use to determine whether they are hazardous. Table 1 provides resources that will aid clinicians in evaluating whether a pharmaceutical agent should be handled as hazardous.

Clinicians should be aware that many drug classifications include medications that are hazardous. Examples of HDs in addition to traditional chemotherapy include thalidomide, interferon alpha, conjugated estrogens, and ganciclovir (NIOSH,

Table 1. Resources for Developing a List of Hazardous Drugs

Resource	Description
American Hospital Formulary Service (AHFS) Pharmacologic-Therapeutic Classification System	The AHFS Pharmacologic-Therapeutic Classification System is a widely accepted system for classification of drugs into categories based on mechanism of action. The system designates all antineoplastic agents as category 10; all category 10 drugs are hazardous.
IARC Monographs on the Evaluation of Carcinogenic Risks to Humans	Monographs categorize the drugs, viruses, and other substances as • Group 1: The agent is carcinogenic to humans. • Group 2A: The agent is probably carcinogenic to humans. • Group 2B: The agent is possibly carcinogenic to humans. • Group 3: The agent is not classifiable as to its carcinogenicity to humans. • Group 4: The agent is probably not carcinogenic to humans.
Material safety data sheets (MSDS)	MSDS are developed by manufacturers to describe the chemical properties of a product, including • Health effects and first aid for exposure • Storage, handling, and disposal information • Personal protection • Procedures for cleaning in the event of a spill. Manufacturers are required to provide MSDS for all drugs that are deemed hazardous or contain hazardous components.
National Toxicology Program's Report on Carcinogens	Carcinogens listed in this report are classified either as known human carcinogens or reasonably anticipated to be human carcinogens. The report can be obtained at http://ntp.niehs.nih.gov/go/roc.
NIOSH	Appendix A of *Preventing Occupational Exposure to Antineoplastic and Other Hazardous Drugs in Health Care Settings* contains a table with a sample list of drugs that should be handled as hazardous. The hazardous drug list was updated in 2010 and can be found at www.cdc.gov/niosh/docs/2010-167/pdfs/2010-167.pdf.
Package inserts for specific pharmaceutical agents	Package inserts for all U.S. Food and Drug Administration–approved medications contain information to assist clinicians in determining whether a drug should be classified as hazardous, including • Drug classification • Pregnancy category and reproductive toxicity • Organ toxicities • Secondary cancers that may develop with exposure • Drug warnings.

Note. Based on information from American Society of Health-System Pharmacists, 2010; International Agency for Research on Cancer, 2006; National Institute for Occupational Safety and Health, 2004; U.S. Department of Health and Human Services, Public Health Service, National Toxicology Program, 2010.

2004). Because HDs are administered in multiple clinical areas, it is imperative that safe handling training extend beyond the oncology unit. HD safe handling is an organizational issue.

Adverse Effects of Hazardous Drug Exposure

The adverse effects of HDs in treated patients are well known and generally seen as outweighed by the benefits of treatment, and measures are implemented to prevent or minimize these hazardous effects. The adverse effects of occupational exposure to HDs in HCWs, on the other hand, have no associated benefit. Precautions that will prevent or minimize occupational exposure to HDs are recommended in the literature. However, despite the existence of published research studies, guidelines, and recommendations, HCWs do not always follow measures to reduce HD exposure. This lack of action places HCWs at risk for myriad adverse effects. Adverse effects of occupational HD exposure are listed by system in Table 2.

Adverse effects of HD exposure can be categorized as either biologic or health effects. The consequences of HD exposure have been reported for more than 30 years. Although biologic effects have not always been linked to changes in health at the time of the studies, those identified have been associated with adverse health outcomes. For example, chemotherapy-related malignancies (myelodysplastic syndrome and acute myeloid leukemia) are known to be associated with specific alterations in chromosomes 5, 7, and 11. These chromosomal changes have occurred in patients receiving alkylating agents for the treatment of cancer.

The following section describes the biologic effects of HDs and is followed by evidence of adverse health outcomes of exposure. Table 3 summarizes studies since 1990 reporting the biologic and health effects of occupational HD exposure.

Biologic Effects of Hazardous Drug Exposure

The most frequently reported biologic effects of occupational HD exposure are genetic damage, chromosomal aberrations, DNA damage, and urinary mutagenicity. Various research studies indicate that nurses who were occupationally exposed to HDs sustained measurable genetic damage, which may be related to increased long-term health effects such as an increased incidence of cancer (Testa et al., 2007). For example, in a recent NIOSH study, the DNA of exposed workers showed a statistically significant increased frequency of damage to chromosome 5 or 7 and an increased frequency of damage to chromosome 5 alone using fluorescence in situ hybridization (McDiarmid, Oliver, Roth, Rogers, & Escalante, 2010).

Deng et al. (2005) found DNA damage, chromosomal damage, and housekeeping gene mutation in 21 workers who were occupationally exposed to methotrexate. These changes were detected by three assays and demonstrated a significant increase compared to unexposed controls. Burgaz et al. (2002) found cyclophosphamide in the urine of nurses, as well as increased genetic damage, following occupational HD handling. The authors emphasized that HD exposure should be kept to a minimum until the long-term effects of chronic low-dose occupational exposure are more fully understood. Not all studies have reported biologic effects of HD exposure, however. Monitoring methods and differences in safe handling precaution use may be an explanation for the different findings.

Adverse Health Outcomes of Occupational Hazardous Drug Exposure

The most frequently reported adverse health outcomes of work-related HD exposure are the occurrence of acute symptoms and reproductive effects. Evidence also has shown an increase in cancer occurrence in occupationally exposed workers.

Table 2. Adverse Health Effects of Occupational Exposure to Hazardous Drugs

System Affected by Hazardous Drug Exposure	Adverse Health Effect of the Exposure
Malignancies	Leukemia Non-Hodgkin lymphoma Bladder cancer Liver cancer
Reproductive	Infertility Prolonged time to conception Premature delivery Low birth weight Ectopic pregnancy Spontaneous abortions; miscarriages Stillbirths Learning disabilities in offspring
Integumentary and mucosal	Skin irritation/contact dermatitis Mouth and nasal sores Hair thinning, partial alopecia
Neurologic	Headaches Dizziness
Gastrointestinal	Nausea Vomiting Abdominal pain
Respiratory	Dyspnea
Allergic	Allergic asthma Eye irritation

Note. Based on information from Fransman, Roeleveld, et al., 2007; Martin, 2005b; Petralia et al., 1999; Saurel-Cubizolles et al., 1993; Skov et al., 1990, 1992; Valanis et al., 1993a, 1999; Walusiak et al., 2002.

Table 3. Hazardous Drug Exposure: Biologic and Health Effects

Study	Purpose	Design	Sample	Measurement	Results
Krepinsky et al., 1990	Evaluate possible genetic damage caused by HD exposure and to compare the effectiveness of three methods of detection	Matched case-controlled	10 exposed and 10 unexposed nurses and 10 patients with cancer receiving chemotherapy in Canada	CAs and SCEs in PBLs. Ames test for mutagenicity in urine. Samples collected before and after exposure. PPE use was not monitored.	SCE assay detected treated patients and 2 nurses who smoked. Ames test detected treated patients but not smokers. CAs detected in 4 out of 9 patients (data missing for 1 patient) and in exposed nurses after several days, which was not likely due to exposure.
Oestreicher et al., 1990	Evaluate possible genetic damage caused by HD exposure	Matched case-controlled	8 nurses handling HDs without protection for years, 8 exposed pharmacy personnel using precautions, 8 unexposed nurses	CAs and SCEs in PBLs	CAs significantly increased in exposed nurses when compared to unexposed nurses and pharmacists using precautions (p < 0.01). SCEs not significantly different between groups.
Stücker et al., 1990	Analyze relationship between SAs and occupational exposure to HDs among nurses	Matched case-controlled	4 French hospitals 466 women, 534 pregnancies	Questionnaire	26% SA in 139 pregnancies in exposed women 15% SA in 357 pregnancies in unexposed women OR = 1.7 (95% CI 1.2–2.8)
Cooke et al., 1991	Determine the occurrence of CAs in nurses and pharmacists exposed to HDs in United Kingdom	Case-controlled	50 pharmacists, 11 nurses, 12 controls, and 6 patients	Analysis of blood for CAs in PBLs	No significant differences between exposed pharmacists or nurses compared to controls No correlation between amount of drugs handled and CAs
Thiringer et al., 1991	Determine the relationship between urine mutagenicity, urinary thioethers, SCEs, and micronuclei and occupational exposure to HDs	Matched case-controlled	60 Swedish nurses exposed to HDs and 60 unexposed controls	Analysis of urine for mutagenicity and thioethers and blood for SCEs and micronuclei in PBLs	For urine mutagenicity, there was a significant difference between exposed and unexposed workers (p < 0.01). For SCEs, there was a significant difference between exposed and unexposed workers (p < 0.05). No significant difference for thioethers and micronuclei
Goloni-Bertollo et al., 1992	Determine the relationship between CAs and SCEs and occupational exposure to HDs	Matched case-controlled	15 nurses and nurse aides in Brazil preparing and administering HDs Controls: 15 nurses on nononcology wards and 15 office workers	Analysis of blood for SCEs and micronuclei in PBLs	Significantly more frequent CAs and SCEs in exposed nurses compared to controls
Harris et al., 1992	Determine the relationship between CAs and micronuclei and occupational exposure to HDs	Matched case-controlled	64 nurses in United States (24 low exposure, 21 medium exposure, 19 high exposure) and 15 patients with cancer	Analysis of blood for CAs and micronuclei in PBLs	No association between exposure classification and CAs or micronuclei CAs and micronuclei significantly associated with glove use of less than 100% of time compared to 100% use

(Continued on next page)

Table 3. Hazardous Drug Exposure: Biologic and Health Effects *(Continued)*

Study	Purpose	Design	Sample	Measurement	Results
Skov et al., 1992	Describe the risk for cancer and adverse reproductive outcomes among Danish nurses handling HDs	Descriptive, retrospective record review	1,282 female nurses from Danish hospitals preparing or administering HDs and 2,572 unexposed nurses working in the same hospitals	Danish health records (1973–1987) Hospital employment records	Significantly increased relative risk for leukemia. Overall risk estimates were not increased for adverse reproductive outcomes. The study included the time before as well as the time after implementation of safe handling measures.
Stücker et al., 1993	Determine the relationship between birth weight and exposure to HDs during and before pregnancy	Matched case-controlled	4 French hospitals 466 women; 420 live births, 298 births to unexposed women, 107 births to nurses exposed during and before pregnancy	Questionnaire	Birth weight of infants of exposed mothers was 85 g less than that of infants of unexposed mothers but was not statistically significant. Exposure data missing for 15.
Valanis et al., 1993a	Determine the relationship between occupational exposure to HDs and acute symptoms among nursing personnel	Descriptive, cross-sectional	1,932 nurses and 152 nurse aides from more than 200 healthcare facilities currently handling HDs	Questionnaire (handling activities, use of PPE, and symptoms experienced in the previous three months)	Handling HDs increased the number of symptoms. Use of protection decreased the number of reported symptoms. Skin contact while cleaning up spills or handling patient excreta was a predictor of symptoms.
Valanis et al., 1993b	Determine the relationship between occupational exposure to HDs and acute symptoms among pharmacy personnel	Descriptive, cross-sectional	533 pharmacists and technicians currently handling HDs and 205 pharmacists and technicians who never mixed HDs	Questionnaire (handling activities, use of PPE, and symptoms in the previous three months)	Diarrhea and chronic cough were increased in exposed study subjects over controls. Self-reported skin contact was a predictor of symptoms.
Hansen & Olsen, 1994	Determine cancer incidence among HD handlers	Archived data analysis	Female Danish pharmacy technicians identified in cancer registry	Comparison of Danish cancer registry data to expected cancer incidence rates	1.5-fold elevated risk of nonmelanoma skin cancer; 3.7-fold increased risk for non-Hodgkin lymphoma
Sessink et al., 1994	Compare urinary CP excretion and CAs in four groups of hospital workers with various levels of HD exposure	Descriptive	17 Dutch and 11 Czech hospital workers handling HDs, and 35 Dutch and 23 Czech workers not handling HDs	Analysis of urine for CP and blood for CAs in PBLs	The percentage of aberrant cells was increased in exposed Dutch and Czech workers. Results suggest additive effect of exposure and smoking. CP was detected in urine samples of 3 out of 11 Dutch workers and 8 out of 11 Czech workers handling HDs.
Fuchs et al., 1995	Determine the occurrence of DNA damage in nurses handling antineoplastic agents	Descriptive	91 nurses from four hospitals in Germany who handled chemotherapy and 54 unexposed controls	Blood samples for DNA single-strand breaks and alkali labile sites in PBLs Questionnaire and demographic data	A 50% higher level of DNA strand breaks and alkali labile sites were detected in nurses not using precautions as compared to controls. After implementing recommended safety precautions, strand breaks decreased to the level of controls.

(Continued on next page)

PAGE 8　　　　　　　　SAFE HANDLING OF HAZARDOUS DRUGS, SECOND EDITION

Table 3. Hazardous Drug Exposure: Biologic and Health Effects *(Continued)*

Study	Purpose	Design	Sample	Measurement	Results
Oesch et al., 1995	Determine the occurrence of DNA damage in nurses handling HDs	Case-controlled	German nurses handling HDs without proper safety equipment, nurses handling HDs with proper equipment, and unexposed controls	DNA strand breaks in PBLs	DNA strand breaks were greater in nurses without proper equipment compared to those with proper equipment ($p < 0.005$) and greater than in unexposed controls
Sessink et al., 1995	Calculate cancer risk for healthcare workers occupationally exposed to CP	Mathematical calculation	Data from an animal study Dose-response data on primary and secondary tumors in CP-treated patients Data on urinary excretion of CP	Dose-response data Estimated mean total CP uptake	For a 70 kg (154 pound) person working 200 days per year for 40 years: cancer risks obtained from both animal and patient data were the same and ranged from 1.4–10 per million per year for CP exposure.
Shortridge et al., 1995	Determine whether HD handling increases the prevalence of menstrual dysfunction in nurses	Descriptive	982 ONS members who handled HDs and 897 ANA members not exposed to HDs All were menstruating, non-pregnant females 46 years of age or younger	Questionnaire	Menstrual dysfunction differed among exposure groups, with the highest rate among study subjects currently handling HDs. Menstrual dysfunction was greatest for study subjects older than age 30.
Valanis et al., 1997	Analyze the relationship between infertility and occupational exposure to HDs among nurses and pharmacists	Descriptive, matched case-controlled	405 subjects reporting infertility and 1,215 matched controls	Questionnaire	Women had a significantly elevated OR (1.5, 95% CI) for infertility associated with HD handling prior to onset of infertility. A similar effect was found in men.
Garaj-Vrhovac & Kopjar, 1998	Determine the relationship between micronuclei and occupational exposure to HDs using three types of staining methods	Matched case-controlled	10 Croatian nurses exposed to HDs and 10 unexposed without adequate protection when preparing and administering HDs	Analysis of blood for micronuclei in PBLs	With the three staining methods, there was a significant difference between the exposed and controls ($p < 0.05$).
Labuhn et al., 1998	Analyze internal and external exposure to HDs	Descriptive	23 pharmacists who prepared HDs, 28 nurses who prepared and administered HDs, 32 nurses who administered HDs, and 35 controls who never handled HDs	Drug-handling log, 24-hour urine for mutagenicity, industrial hygiene (fluorescent) scans for doxorubicin contamination	15% of the urine samples were positive for mutagenicity; reported skin exposure predicted positive urine tests. 13% of scans were positive for worker contamination. More contamination occurred during HD administration than during preparation. Reported PPE use was 27% among nurses who handled HDs.
Valanis et al., 1999	Determine the effect of HD exposure on pregnancy loss among nurses and pharmacists	Descriptive	7,094 pregnancies among 2,976 pharmacy and nursing staff	Questionnaire	Exposure of the mother to HDs directly before or during pregnancy was associated with a significantly increased risk of SA and/or stillbirth.

(Continued on next page)

Table 3. Hazardous Drug Exposure: Biologic and Health Effects *(Continued)*

Study	Purpose	Design	Sample	Measurement	Results
Maluf & Erdtmann, 2000	Part 1: Analyze the relationship between micronuclei and occupational exposure to HDs among nurses and pharmacists	Matched case-controlled	10 Brazilian pharmacists and nurses exposed to HDs and 10 unexposed workers	Analysis of blood for micronuclei in PBLs	Significant difference between exposed workers and controls (p = 0.038)
	Part 2: Analyze the relationship between micronuclei and comet assay and modifications to work schedules among nurses and pharmacists	Matched case-controlled following reduction in work hours	12 Brazilian pharmacists and nurses exposed to HDs and 12 controls	Analysis of blood for micronuclei and comet assay in PBLs	No difference between exposed workers and controls for micronuclei Significant difference between exposed workers and controls for comet assay (p = 0.0006)
Burgaz et al., 2002	Determine frequency of CAs in PBLs of nurses exposed to HDs	Matched case-controlled	20 nurses handling HDs and 18 controls	CAs in PBL; CP excreted in urine	2.5-fold increase in CAs, including chromatid breaks, gaps, and acentric fragments for nurses handling HDs as compared to controls (p < 0.05) CP excretion rate for 12 nurses was 1.63 mcg/24 hours, indicating exposure.
Cavallo et al., 2005	Evaluate genotoxic effects of antineoplastic exposure	Laboratory analysis	25 exposed nurses, 5 pharmacy technicians, and 30 unexposed controls from administrative offices in a large Italian hospital	Micronuclei test and analysis of CAs with lymphocytes and exfoliated buccal cells	No difference between exposed study subjects and controls for micronuclei in lymphocytes Higher values for micronuclei in exfoliated buccal cells of exposed workers CAs were 2.5–5-fold higher in exposed groups.
Martin, 2005b	Determine the effects of chemotherapy handling among nurses and their offspring	Descriptive, correlational	2,427 nurses who reported handling 3 or more doses of HDs per day for at least one year and reported giving birth within 10 years of exposure Total of 3,399 offspring	Questionnaire	HD handling before age 25 increased odds of infertility. More years of HD handling resulted in higher rate of miscarriage. Handling 9 or more doses per day increased preterm labor and preterm birth. Learning disabilities increased in offspring of nurses who rarely wore gloves during HD handling. Increased cancer occurrence existed among exposed nurses.
Yoshida et al., 2006	Analyze the relationship between DNA damage and occupational HD exposure in nurses and pharmacists	Case-controlled	37 nurses in a hospital in Japan: 18 unexposed and 19 exposed nurses	Analysis of blood for comet assay, tail length	Tail length, 5.1 mcm in unexposed and 8.5 mcm in exposed study subjects Significant difference, p = 0.004

(Continued on next page)

Table 3. Hazardous Drug Exposure: Biologic and Health Effects *(Continued)*

Study	Purpose	Design	Sample	Measurement	Results
Fransman, Roeleveld, et al., 2007	Determine reproductive effects of HD exposure	Survey	4,393 exposed and unexposed nurses	Estimated HD exposure based on self-reported tasks Reproductive outcomes	Nurses highly exposed to HDs took longer to conceive than unexposed nurses. Exposure was associated with premature delivery and low birth weight.
Ikeda et al., 2007	Analyze the relationship between SCEs and occupational exposure to HDs among mixed population Determine epirubicin in urine and plasma of mixed population	Case-controlled; laboratory analysis	Pharmacists, nurses, and physicians in Japan with rotating duties SCE: 11 exposed workers and 2 controls Urine and plasma analysis: 13 exposed workers and 3 controls	SCEs in peripheral blood Epirubicin in urine and plasma	No correlation was found between hours worked per week and SCEs. No epirubicin was detected in urine or plasma.
Testa et al., 2007	Determine the incidence of CAs in PBLs of nurses occupationally exposed to HDs	Case-controlled	76 oncology nurses occupationally exposed to HDs and 72 controls from two hospitals in Italy	CAs in PBLs	Mean total number of CAs for exposed nurses was 3.7 times (11.2 versus 3.04) that of controls ($p < 0.0001$). Chromatid- and chromosome-type aberrations were 3.4 and 4.16 times that of controls.

ANA—American Nurses Association; CA—chromosomal aberration; CI—confidence interval; CP—cyclophosphamide; DNA—deoxyribonucleic acid; HD—hazardous drug; ONS—Oncology Nursing Society; OR—odds ratio; PBLs—peripheral blood lymphocytes; PPE—personal protective equipment; SA—spontaneous abortion; SCE—sister chromatid exchanges

Several studies have documented the adverse reproductive outcomes of occupational exposure. Fransman, Roeleveld, et al. (2007) compared outcomes in 4,393 exposed and unexposed (control) nurses in the Netherlands. Exposure to antineoplastic drugs was estimated using dermal measurements based on handling tasks. Nurses who were highly exposed, defined as 0.74 mcg/week exposure, took longer to conceive, had infants with lower birth weight, and had a higher incidence of preterm labor. Similarly, Martin (2005b) reported an inverse relationship between compliance with HD handling guidelines and adverse reproductive outcomes among nurses surveyed. Significant findings in exposed versus unexposed nurses included infertility in those who handled chemotherapy before age 25; miscarriages, preterm birth, and preterm labor in nurses who administered more than nine doses per day; and an increase in learning disabilities in offspring, which correlated to glove use. When a Danish study of exposed versus unexposed nurses found a similar risk of fetal malformations, miscarriages, low birth weight, or preterm delivery, the researchers concluded that a well-protected setting (e.g., one with proper safe handling precautions) reduces occupational HD exposure (Skov et al., 1992).

Valanis, Vollmer, Labuhn, and Glass (1993a) reported the occurrence of acute symptoms of HD exposure in 2,084 nurses and nurse aides. These included cardiac, gastrointestinal, neurologic, allergic, infectious, and systemic symptoms. The researchers found that skin contact with HDs, especially during spill cleanup, was associated with less use of personal protective equipment (PPE) and more acute symptoms, leading the authors to conclude that skin contact is a major source of exposure.

Several studies have found an increase in the occurrence of cancer in HD-exposed HCWs compared to unexposed HCWs. For instance, Skov et al. (1992) found a higher relative risk for acute leukemia in female Danish nurses handling chemotherapy. Hansen and Olsen (1994) reported that long-term pharmacy dispensers of HDs were 3.7 times more likely than the general population to develop non-Hodgkin lymphoma. Martin (2005b) found that HD-exposed nurses had a higher occurrence of cancer and that the cancer occurred at a younger age than expected according to National Cancer Institute (NCI) Surveillance, Epidemiology, and End Results data.

Recent studies document genetic changes in HD handlers and fewer acute side effects experienced by HD-exposed HCWs when compared to earlier studies. This is likely due to both improved use of safe handling precautions and the availability of more sensitive measures of HD exposure. The effects of low-dose, chronic HD exposure are not well documented, but several recognized consequences of exposure exist. While overall exposure is lower than in years past, HCWs are still potentially exposed. Publications from around the world indicate that adherence to HD safe handling guidelines is lower than what is recommended. Nurses must recognize deficiencies in their systems, individual practices, and PPE use and make corrections to avoid the adverse biologic and health effects of HD exposure.

Evidence for Occupational Hazardous Drug Exposure

Occupational HD exposure is not as easy to measure as radiation exposure. In clinical settings, workers who have the potential for radiation exposure wear a film badge or dosimeter that records exposure as it occurs. The measuring devices are evaluated on a regular basis, and the HCW is notified when a predetermined level of exposure is exceeded. Individuals are counseled to then avoid exposure for a period of time. Currently, no reliable method exists for biologic monitoring of occupational exposure to HDs (Baker & Connor, 1996). Several methods (Ames test, sister chromatid exchanges, chromosomal aberrations, micronucleus assay, and urinary thioether excretion) have been found to correlate poorly with HD exposure. For this and other reasons, no recommendations have been made for routine testing for HD exposure.

Biologic Monitoring

HD exposure in HCWs occurs through various routes, including dermal absorption, absorption through mucous membranes, and inadvertent ingestion, inhalation, or injection. When HD exposure occurs, the drugs are absorbed, metabolized, and excreted. Assays have been developed for directly measuring specific HDs or their metabolites. Detecting these drugs in the urine of HCWs is one method of determining HD exposure.

In three studies by Sessink and colleagues, urine samples were analyzed using sensitive and specific high-performance liquid chromatography and gas chromatography-mass spectrometry (Sessink, Boer, Scheefhals, Anzion, & Bos, 1992; Sessink, Van de Kerkhof, Anzion, Noordhoek, & Bos, 1994; Sessink, Wittenhorst, Anzion, & Bos, 1997). HDs were detected in the urine of workers, including workers not directly involved in preparation or administration of the specific drugs. The authors concluded that routine handling of HDs results in contamination of the work environment and that dermal exposure is an important route for uptake of these drugs. This is supported by an earlier report that detected cyclophosphamide both in the urine of volunteers who had the drug applied to their skin and in two nurses who prepared and administered cyclophosphamide without respiratory protection or PPE (Hirst, Tse, Mills, Levin, & White, 1984).

Additional studies using assays indicated exposure, uptake, and metabolism of HDs during routine work activities even when no obvious source of exposure was identified. Nygren and Lundgren (1997) detected increased platinum (from platinum-containing HDs such as cisplatin) in the blood of staff nurses (those involved in patient care) but not in graduate nurses (those involved in HD handling) or pharmacists. They concluded that exposure most likely occurred during routine care of treated patients rather than during HD preparation or administration, where PPE use was more likely. Pethran et al. (2003) found HDs in the urine of 40% of study participants despite the use of biologic safety cabinets (BSCs).

Environmental Monitoring for Hazardous Drug Exposure

Early support for precautions while handling HDs focused on the biologic effects in exposed individuals. Following the implementation of HD safe handling guidelines in most settings, pharmacists and nurses continued to demonstrate evidence of exposure despite the use of precautions such as BSCs, gloves, and gowns. The most plausible source of exposure is an environment that is contaminated with HDs.

Exposure From Contaminated Surfaces

One method of measuring environmental contamination with HDs is surface wipe sampling. Surfaces in work areas where HDs are handled are evaluated for the presence of HD residue. The sample areas are measured, moistened with 0.03 M sodium hydroxide, and wiped with paper towels until dry. The towels are placed in plastic containers and sent for analysis for the presence of several drugs (Connor, Anderson, Sessink, & Spivey, 2002).

Minoia et al. (1998) analyzed surface wipe samples, pads placed on gowns, air samples, and gloves of 24 workers involved in HD preparation and administration for the presence of cyclophosphamide and ifosfamide. In addition to positive air and urine samples, many of the wipe samples taken from inside and outside of the BSC, including the floor and door handles, were contaminated with the two drugs. Many of the pads and gloves were also contaminated. The authors concluded that inadequate performance of the BSC may result in worker contamination. They suggested that using a plastic-backed paper liner inside the BSC may interfere with airflow and affect BSC performance. No subsequent studies have evaluated the effect of BSC liners on airflow. The study further demonstrated that gloves are routinely contaminated during HD handling and should be changed periodically. Guidelines recommend that gloves be discarded after no more than 30 minutes of use.

In a multisite study in the United States and Canada, surface contamination with three cytotoxic agents was measured by more than 200 wipe samples (Connor, Anderson, Sessink, Broadfield, & Power, 1999). The results revealed that 75% of wipe samples from drug preparation areas and 65% of samples from drug administration areas had measurable levels of one or more of the drugs. The investigators concluded that surface contamination with HDs is common and that workers who are not directly involved in HD handling may be exposed to drug residue on these surfaces. Other investigators have reported similar findings with cyclophosphamide (Kiffmeyer et al., 2002) and platinum (from cisplatin and/or carboplatin) in addition to ifosfamide (Mason et al., 2005; Nygren & Aspman, 2004; Schmaus, Schierl, & Funck, 2002).

Fransman, Vermeulen, and Kromhout (2004, 2005) evaluated workers' potential and actual dermal exposure to cyclophosphamide during the performance of common hospital tasks in two studies. The investigators placed pads on several body locations of nurses, pharmacy technicians, and cleaning personnel. They also analyzed gloves worn during handling activities, hand-wash water used after handling activities, patient body fluids, and linens from patients who had received cyclophosphamide. The gloves were commonly contaminated. Nurses were found to have skin contamination under gloves, especially following handling of patients' urine. These findings confirmed dermal exposure during normal patient care activities and led the authors to conclude that hands are a common site of HD exposure for HCWs.

Several studies have detected drug contamination on the outside of drug vials when delivered by the manufacturers (Connor et al., 2005; Nygren, Gustavsson, Strom, & Friberg, 2002; Sessink et al., 1992). Cyclophosphamide, fluorouracil, ifosfamide, and platinum have all been detected on vial exteriors using various wipe sampling and washing techniques. These findings indicate that nurses and pharmacists are at risk for skin exposure if they do not wear PPE while handling unopened drug vials.

Results from the many environmental monitoring studies demonstrate that the work areas where HDs are prepared and administered are commonly contaminated with the drugs. Workers who normally wear PPE for direct drug-handling activities can be exposed when touching unknowingly contaminated surfaces with unprotected hands. Every study measuring environmental contamination using surface wipe sampling found evidence of surface contamination (see Table 4).

Inhalation Exposure

Several investigators have identified low levels of HDs in air samples collected in areas where the drugs are handled (Kiffmeyer et al., 2002; Kromhout et al., 2000; Mason et al., 2005). Although this exposure route is less likely for workers who use a BSC, the risk is high for drug preparation outside of a primary engineering control (PEC), including inhalation of aerosols during the crushing of tablets (Dorr & Alberts, 1992). In addition, some authors have reported vaporization of several antineoplastic drugs (Connor, Shults, & Fraser, 2000; Kiffmeyer et al., 2002). A few authors have proposed that inhalation exposure may be higher than previously thought because earlier methods used to measure air samples were not sufficiently sensitive (Hedmer, Jonsson, & Nygren, 2004; Larson, Khazaeli, & Dillon, 2003b). Therefore, workers should consider inhalation as a possible route of HD exposure and avoid performing any drug preparation activities outside of a BSC.

To summarize, ongoing evidence shows that occupational HD exposure can and does occur. Few laboratories in the United States perform the assays described in this section, which makes routine monitoring impractical. In the absence of measured contamination in the workplace, nurses should consider the possibility of environmental contamination. Because a safe level of HD exposure does not exist, HCWs must take steps to minimize their exposure. Additional studies are needed that evaluate the magnitude of HD exposure of HCWs who consistently use safe handling precautions.

Table 4. Hazardous Drug Exposure: Environmental Monitoring

Study	Purpose	Design	Sample	Measurement	Results
Sessink et al., 1992	Measure surface contamination and air concentrations with 4 HDs	Laboratory studies	Pharmacy and nursing areas in a hospital in the Netherlands	Analysis of air samples and wipe samples for CP, IF, 5-FU, and MTX	Floors, hood, drug vials, sinks, cleaned urinals, gloves, and other objects > LOD for one or more HD. CP or IF detected in urine of 8 of 25 pharmacy technicians and nurses, including 6 not directly involved in handling.
McDevitt et al., 1993	Measure surface contamination and air concentrations with HDs	Laboratory studies	Pharmacy and nursing areas in a U.S. hospital 76 wipe samples and 73 air samples	Analysis of air samples and wipe samples for CP	Pharmacy, 34 wipe samples, 18% > LOD; air samples, 3/34 > LOD Nursing, 42 wipe samples, 14% > LOD; air samples, 0 of 39 > LOD
Minoia et al., 1998	Evaluate the occupational exposure of hospital personnel handling HDs	Laboratory studies	10 workers involved in HD preparation and 14 workers involved in administration of CP and IF in 2 Italian hospitals	Analysis of air samples, wipe samples, pads, and gloves Urinary excretion of CP and IF measured using HPLC/tandem mass spectrometry	Urine samples were positive for 12 of 24 workers for CP and 2 of 24 workers for IF. 3 of 24 air samples were positive, and wipe samples of surfaces as well as gloves were positive. A plastic-backed liner in the BSC was shown to compromise its containment properties.
Connor et al., 1999	Measure surface contamination with 3 HDs in pharmacy and nursing areas	Laboratory studies	More than 200 locations, including pharmacies and HD administration areas	Surface wipe samples analyzed for IF, CP, and 5-FU Duplicate blanks prepared for every surface sample.	75% of samples from drug preparation areas and 65% of samples from drug administration areas had measurable levels of HDs.
Rubino et al., 1999	Measure surface contamination with 4 HDs in pharmacy areas	Laboratory studies	8 oncology departments in 2 Italian hospitals	139 surface wipe samples for MTX, 5-FU, cytarabine, and gemcitabine measured at various distances from drug preparation area	Percent of samples with contamination: 83% > LOD in safety cabinet 53% > LOD < 1 M from safety cabinet 47% > LOD > 1 M from safety cabinet
Kromhout et al., 2000	Evaluate the potential for dermal exposure to HDs	Observation, simulation, and laboratory studies	Patient treatment areas in 3 hospitals in the Netherlands	Visual scoring of fluorescent tracer found on workers and work surfaces Air sampling for airborne particles of HDs using gas chromatography/tandem mass spectrometry	Leakage detected at connection sites of IV equipment. Leakage highest at the IV spike connection and lowest at Luer-lock connections. Floors, toilets, and soles of nurses' shoes were contaminated. CP was found in 16% of samples taken in patient treatment areas.

(Continued on next page)

Table 4. Hazardous Drug Exposure: Environmental Monitoring *(Continued)*

Study	Purpose	Design	Sample	Measurement	Results
Favier et al., 2001	Measure environmental contamination with HDs in BSCs and isolators	Laboratory analysis	6 French pharmacies, 3 with BSCs and 3 with isolators	Measurement of 5-FU on work surfaces in BSCs and isolators and several other locations	Comparable samples from the 3 BSCs, 1 of 6 > LOD. Samples from isolators, 5 of 6 > LOD. Values post-cleaning were lower. 25 of 30 preps in isolator > LOD. 1 of 30 preps in BSCs > LOD. Some other glove and environmental contamination was reported.
Kiffmeyer et al., 2002	Measure environmental contamination with HDs	Laboratory analysis	HD preparation areas	Measurement of carmustine, cisplatin, CP, etoposide, and 5-FU in air samples. Measurement of CP in wipe samples and urine of workers who prepared CP.	Particulate CP was found in the air of 6 of 20 preparation sites. Gaseous CP was found in 7 of 15 sites. CP was present on 17 of 26 surfaces. No CP was found in the urine of 3 tested workers.
Nygren et al., 2002	Measure external vial contamination with HDs	Laboratory analysis	6 vials of platinum-containing drugs from 3 different manufacturers in Sweden	Wipe sample analysis using adsorptive voltammetry	Drug vials were contaminated on the outside when delivered by the manufacturer.
Schmaus et al., 2002	Measure environmental contamination with HDs	Laboratory analysis	7 standard locations in each of 14 hospital pharmacies in Germany	Wipe sample analysis using gas chromatography-mass spectrometry and voltammetry for CP, IF, 5-FU, and platinum	100% of samples tested positive for platinum, which has a low limit of detection. 0%–25% tested positive for CP and IF; 40%–80% tested positive for 5-FU. Volume of drugs prepared did not predict the amount of contamination. Work practices in some settings reduced contamination.
Favier et al., 2003	Measure external vial contamination	Laboratory analysis	739 vials tested for 6 drugs from several manufacturers. Drug packaging tested for 5-FU and etoposide	Vials immersed in solvent with rotation for 30 seconds in water. HPLC used for 5-FU, etoposide, doxorubicin, and docetaxel. Gas chromatography used for CP and IF	100% of vials were contaminated 0.5–2,447 ng/vial. 5-FU drug packaging was contaminated. No contamination was seen on etoposide packaging.
Larson et al., 2003a	Method development	Laboratory analysis	Development of a method for detecting 5-FU, IF, CP, doxorubicin, and paclitaxel in air samples	Air samples collected and filtered with Anasorb® 708 (SKC, Inc.) solid sorbent tube	Greater than 90% recovery for both CP and ifosfamide; 5-FU, doxorubicin, and paclitaxel were detected and measured. All 5 agents of interest were detected at minimal LOD of 0.5 mcg/ml.

(Continued on next page)

Table 4. Hazardous Drug Exposure: Environmental Monitoring (Continued)

Study	Purpose	Design	Sample	Measurement	Results
Larson et al., 2003b	Validate a new monitoring method for evaluation of airborne HDs	Laboratory analysis	Filters and sorbent tubes used for recovering CP, IF, and 5-FU from air samples	Air monitoring for HDs using reverse-phase HPLC/mass spectrometry	CP was recovered from filters and then evaporated, becoming gaseous. HEPA filters trap particles but not vapors. Recirculating BSCs may result in worker exposure.
Fransman et al., 2004	Evaluate dermal exposure to CP	Laboratory analysis	Pharmacy technicians, oncology nurses, and cleaning personnel in 3 Dutch hospitals during the performance of 5 tasks	Analysis of cotton pads attached to body surfaces. Analysis of wipe samples of foreheads. Assays of used gloves, wash water, wash cloths, towels, and bed-sheets for CP	CP was detected on pads, gloves, wipe samples, wash cloths, and bed linens. CP was found on foreheads of technicians and nurses. Cleaning personnel had CP on their gloves. Contamination of hand-wash samples was highest during handling of urine.
Hedmer et al., 2004	Validation of methods for detecting CP on surfaces and in the air	Laboratory analysis	Air and surface samples	Wipes made of different materials to clean up CP. Several filter types for recovering CP from air	LOD for CP was 0.02 ng per sample for wipes and 0.03 ng for air samples.
Nygren & Aspman, 2004	Validation of x-ray fluorescence as a method for assessment of aerosol distribution	Laboratory analysis	Surfaces in a drug preparation room of an oncology clinic	Wipe samples analyzed for platinum	Platinum was recovered from every wipe sample except from a corridor outside the preparation room. The level of platinum was highest in the BSC and decreased with increasing distance from the BSC.
Connor et al., 2005	3 studies evaluating external vial contamination with HDs	Laboratory analysis	Unopened vials of HDs	Study 1: wipe sampling for CP and IF. Study 2: wipe sampling for CP and 5-FU. Study 3: analysis for cisplatin using two vial washing techniques and polymer sleeves	Surface contamination was detected on most commercially available drug vials tested. Improved decontamination in combination with sleeves reduced contamination by 90%.
Fransman et al., 2005	Measure dermal exposure to CP during various handling activities	Laboratory analysis	Personnel handling HDs or caring for people who receive HDs	Analysis of cotton pads attached to body surfaces. Analysis of wipe samples of foreheads. Assays of used gloves, wash water, wash cloths, towels, and bed-sheets for CP	CP was detected on pads, gloves, wipe samples, wash cloths, and bed linens. Most CP was found on hands. Nurses who wore gloves had skin contamination of their hands, most often after handling urine.

(Continued on next page)

Table 4. Hazardous Drug Exposure: Environmental Monitoring (Continued)

Study	Purpose	Design	Sample	Measurement	Results
Mason et al., 2005	Evaluate the effectiveness of negative and positive pressure isolators	Laboratory analysis	Air, urine, and surface samples from two hospital pharmacies in the United Kingdom	Analysis of air samples and urine samples Surface wipe sample to measure floor and glove contamination	Measurable amounts of HDs were detected on floors and on gloves of staff preparing HDs. Low levels of platinum were found in the urine, with significantly higher amounts in workers using negative pressure isolators. Personal air samples were mostly undetectable.
Zeedijk et al., 2005	Method development	Laboratory analysis	Method development for detecting residue of CP, IF, 5-FU, and MTX, pre- and post-cleaning of surfaces	Wipe samples tested using HPLC for 5-FU TDx FLx Immunology Analyzer for MTX Gas chromatography/mass spectrometry for CP and IF	4 drugs can be measured from one wipe sample. Pre-cleaning over 3 days, 15 of 15 > LOD Post-cleaning over 3 days, 10 of 14 > LOD
Bussieres et al., 2007	Measure environmental contamination with HDs	Laboratory study	Develop method for measuring MTX in a Canadian pharmacy	MTX from wipe samples using HPLC over 40 sampling times	5 of 198 wipe samples > LOD
Fransman, Huizer, et al., 2007	Measure environmental contamination with HDs	Laboratory study	Measurement of 8 drugs in air and on gloves, hands, and bed linens in a Dutch laundry	Air sample collected in linen handling area Linen strips and gloves tested for 8 drugs using triple quadruple mass spectrometer	Before pre-wash, 5 of 15 sheets > LOD 3, CP; 2, IF; 1, 5-FU After pre-wash, 0 of 15 > LOD
Ikeda et al., 2007	Measure environmental contamination with HDs	Laboratory study	Develop method for measuring epirubicin in a Japanese pharmacy	Wipe samples measured from 11 different surfaces with HPLC	14 of 59 > LOD

BSC—biologic safety cabinet; CP—cyclophosphamide; 5-FU—fluorouracil; HD—hazardous drug; HEPA—high-efficiency particulate air; HPLC—high-performance liquid chromatography; IF—ifosfamide; LOD—level of detection; MTX—methotrexate

Hierarchy of Controls

Introduction

OSHA defines *industrial hygiene* as "the science of anticipating, recognizing, evaluating, and controlling workplace conditions that may cause workers' injury or illness" (OSHA, 1998).

The principles of industrial hygiene apply to the safe handling of hazardous agents, including HDs. As substitution of nonhazardous drugs is not an option, the recognized methods of decreasing employee exposure to HDs are by implementing engineering, work practice, and administrative controls (see Figure 1).

Engineering controls reduce worker exposure at the source by eliminating the hazard or by isolating the worker from the hazard. Engineering controls include machines and equipment that are designed to either contain the hazard or provide appropriate ventilation. When engineering controls do not eliminate the risk, PPE must be added to provide barrier protection from the hazard. Specific work practices that change the way work is performed may effectively reduce worker exposure. Administrative controls reduce workers' exposure by establishing appropriate, and mandatory, work procedures; restricting access to potentially contaminated areas; and scheduling risky tasks so that the fewest employees are exposed. This section will discuss how the hierarchy of controls applies to HD handling in the healthcare environment.

Figure 1. Hierarchy of Controls

Most effective → (arrow pointing up)

- Elimination of the hazard
- Engineering controls
- Administrative controls
- Work practice controls

Least effective

- Personal protective equipment

Note. Based on information from Occupational Safety and Health Administration, 1998.

Engineering Controls

Engineering controls for compounding sterile HD doses must be designed to protect the sterility of the drug and to provide containment of drug residue generated during the compounding process. The United States Pharmacopeia (USP) is a public standards–setting authority for medicines and healthcare products manufactured or sold in the United States. The USP sets standards for the "quality, purity, strength, and consistency" of drugs and solutions (USP, n.d., para. 1). USP General Chapter 797, "Pharmaceutical Compounding—Sterile Preparations," addresses the standards for the compounding of sterile preparations (USP, 2008a). The USP uses the term *primary engineering control*, or PEC, to describe devices that provide a clean environment for compounding sterile drugs. A clean air environment is accomplished by filtering air through high-efficiency particulate air (HEPA) filters. The quality of the air is measured by the number of particles per cubic meter; the lower the particulate count, the cleaner the compounding environment. The International Organization for Standardization (ISO, 1999) rates the environment based on the particle count, with a lower ISO class number indicating a cleaner environment. An ISO Class 5 environment is required for compounding sterile IV drugs (USP, 2008a). USP 797 also addresses the special requirements for HD preparation (see Figure 2).

NIOSH (2004), in its alert on HDs, uses the term *ventilated cabinet* to describe the type of engineering control that minimizes worker exposure by containing airborne HD contaminants. For sterile doses of HDs, the appropriate engineering controls include BSCs and compounding aseptic containment isolators (CACIs), as these cabinets provide both product and personnel protection (ASHP, 2006;

Figure 2. U.S. Pharmacopeia Chapter 797 Summary of Requirements for Compounding Hazardous Drugs

HD storage	PEC ISO Class 5	Buffer Area ISO Class 7	Ante Area ISO Class 7
• Shall be separate • Negative pressure preferred • ACPH = 12	• BSC or CACI • Optimally vented 100% to outside • CACI that meets USP 797 requirements may be in negative pressure area with 12 ACPH—no buffer area required	• Shall be separate; NO sink • Optimally negative pressure to ante area • ACPH = 30 • 15 ACPH may come from PEC	• ISO Class 7 or better; sink OK • Positive pressure to buffer area • ACPH = 30

ACPH—air changes per hour; BSC—biologic safety cabinet; CACI—compounding aseptic containment isolator; HD—hazardous drug; ISO—International Organization for Standardization; PEC—primary engineering control

Note. Based on information from U.S. Pharmacopeia, 2008a.

NIOSH, 2004; USP, 2008a). Compounding of nonsterile doses of HDs or other activities where containment ventilation is desired may be done in a non–ISO Class 5 ventilated environment, such as a fume hood (Class I BSC). If nonsterile activities are done in the ISO Class 5 PEC, full decontamination for HD residue and cleaning and disinfection for particulates are required prior to resuming sterile compounding (Controlled Environment Testing Association [CETA], 2007). It must be recognized that PECs do not eliminate the generation of contamination and may have limitations in their containment.

Biologic Safety Cabinets

The Class II BSC was adopted in the early 1980s as a valuable tool in reducing occupational exposure while compounding sterile doses of HDs. Originally designed to handle biologics in a laboratory setting, the Class II BSC has HEPA-filtered, vertical-flow unidirectional air supply in the work area of the cabinet, creating the necessary ISO Class 5 compounding environment. It has a glass shield extending across the front of the cabinet with a front opening of 8–10 inches, through which the operator accesses the work area. Inward airflow through this opening combines with the downward airflow and is removed from the work area through front and rear grills. The front air barrier is designed to create a protective air curtain containing contamination generated in the work area within the cabinet. The mixed contaminated air is either recirculated within the cabinet or exhausted to the workroom or outside environment through HEPA filters. The type of cabinet (A1, A2, B1, or B2) is determined by the percentage of air that is recirculated and the amount exhausted. The B cabinets exhaust most or all of the contaminated air through outside ventilation and are considered the most effective cabinets in providing environmental and worker protection, especially for HDs that are vaporous. HEPA filters are not effective for containing volatile materials because they do not capture vapors and gases (National Institutes of Health, 1994). NIOSH (2004) recommends to not use a recirculating cabinet and to exhaust all contaminated air to the outside through HEPA filters and a ducted connection. USP 797 states that the BSC optimally should be 100% vented to the outside air through a HEPA filter (USP, 2008a).

The Class II BSC must meet the performance standards of NSF International/American National Standards Institute Standard 49, and manufacturers must test their cabinets to this standard (NSF International/American National Standards Institute, 2009). The containment of the Class II cabinet is dependent on the airflow within the cabinet and the technique of the operator in accessing the work area through the front air barrier. Studies of workplace contamination have shown HD residue on the floor in front of the Class II BSC (Connor et al., 1999; Sessink et al., 1992, 1994, 1997). These studies indicate a limitation in using this cabinet for drug compounding.

The Class II BSC is also designed to be decontaminated by fumigating with a vigorous disinfectant that permeates into the contaminated air plenums of the cabinet. This decontamination is not effective for drug and other chemical residue. Surface decontamination with detergent and physical wiping may be used to remove drug residue from the Class II BSC; however, many of the air plenums are not reachable to accomplish this (ASHP, 1990).

The Class II cabinets should remain on so that the blower operates continuously to prevent any release of drug residue from the contaminated plenums and under the work surface into the workroom. If the BSC must be turned off, it should first be cleaned and the front opening sealed with plastic and tape to prevent any contaminants from escaping. BSCs should be serviced and certified by a qualified technician at least every six months and any time the cabinet is repaired or moved (ASHP, 1990; USP, 2008a).

Class III BSCs also may be used for sterile compounding of HDs because they provide product and environmental protection (ASHP, 2006; NIOSH, 2004). Class III BSCs are totally enclosed with gas-tight construction. The entire cabinet is under negative pressure, and access to the work area for compounding activities is through attached gloves, which limits floor contamination in front of the cabinet. All of the air is HEPA filtered, and outside exhaust is mandatory through a duct with an auxiliary blower. The Class III cabinet has the same limitations on decontamination as the Class II cabinet. The cost of purchasing, installing, and maintaining this type of cabinet generally is prohibitive, and few are used for extemporaneous sterile compounding.

Compounding Aseptic Containment Isolators

The NIOSH alert on HDs and USP 797 allow the use of an isolator as an alternative to a BSC in compounding HDs (NIOSH, 2004; USP, 2008a). Unlike the Class II BSC, however, no uniform design or performance standards exist for isolators used for pharmaceutical compounding. CETA has produced several application guides to help in the selection and use of compounding isolators in healthcare facilities (CETA, 2008). In the absence of standards, manufacturers have produced varying designs and have marketed isolators for the purpose of pharmaceutical compounding with no evidence of effectiveness. One study examining the different isolator designs found extensive differences in the abilities of the various isolators to handle challenges to the airflow that would occur during pharmaceutical compounding (Peters, McKeon, & Weiss, 2007). The authors concluded that the performance of unidirectional-flow isolators supports their use in pharmacy and nursing operations, whereas the performance of turbulent-flow isolators does not (Peters et al., 2007). USP 797 requires the use of unidirectional airflow in a PEC used to compound sterile preparations (USP, 2008a).

The USP 797 revision sets performance standards for isolators used to compound sterile preparations, for compounding aseptic isolators, and for isolators used to compound sterile HD preparations (CACIs) (USP, 2008a). To meet the criteria of USP 797, an isolator must provide isolation from the room and maintain ISO Class 5 air quality within the cabinet during dynamic operating conditions. Air quality must be documented by particle counts during compounding operations and during material transfer in and out of the isolator. Recovery time to ISO Class 5 air in the main chamber must be documented after material is transferred in and out. Work practices must be developed to reduce disruption of the air quality in the isolator and to minimize recovery time.

Buffer Area and Ante Area

To improve the performance of the PEC in maintaining the required air quality, USP 797 mandates that the PEC be placed in a controlled environment with air quality not less than ISO Class 7, a buffer area created with an additional source of HEPA-filtered air (not solely from the PEC) and having adequate air changes per hour (ACPH) (USP, 2008a). Access to the buffer area must be through a second area, the ante area, which provides transition from noncompounding activities to sterile compounding. The ante area for the sterile compounding of HDs also must be ISO Class 7, as the pressure differentials required for HD containment (negative pressure) forces the air into the buffer area to prevent the escape of HD contamination from the compounding environment into the surrounding work area. The HD compounding and storage areas must be separate from other storage and compounding areas and also be within a controlled environment with adequate ACPH and air pressure controls to contain HD contamination generated during handling activities (NIOSH, 2004; USP, 2008a). HDs may be stored in the buffer or ante areas provided that appropriate cleaning and other work practices are in place.

The CACI must meet USP 797 requirements to be exempted from placement in an ISO Class 7 buffer area. These requirements include provision of isolation from the room and maintenance of ISO Class 5 air during dynamic operating conditions; maintenance of ISO Class 5 air quality during compounding operations; and maintenance of ISO Class 5 air during material transfer, with the particle counter probe located as near to the transfer door as possible without obstructing the transfer. CACI manufacturers must provide documentation that the requirements of USP 797 are met if the CACI is not located in an ISO Class 7 environment (USP, 2008a).

If a CACI meets *all* of the aforementioned requirements in USP 797, it is exempt from the requirement of placing it in an ISO Class 7 buffer area (USP, 2008a). For HD compounding, however, the compounding area where the CACI is located must maintain negative pressure and have a minimum of 12 ACPH (USP, 2008a).

Only authorized, trained staff may have access to the buffer area and only after removing all jewelry and cosmetics and properly garbing and washing (USP, 2008a). No eating, drinking, smoking, chewing gum, application of cosmetics, or storage of food should occur in the ante or buffer areas (OSHA, 1995).

Closed-System Drug Transfer Devices

A closed-system drug transfer device (CSTD) is a drug transfer device that mechanically prevents the transfer of environmental contaminants into the system and the escape of hazardous concentrations of drug or vapor from the system (NIOSH, 2004). These devices are engineering controls that can be used in addition to PECs to reduce HD drug escape that occurs during preparation and administration.

Numerous studies have shown that surface contamination with HD residue occurs in areas where drugs are compounded and administered even when PECs are in place (see Table 4). In a landmark study, Connor et al. (1999) sampled work surfaces in six cancer treatment centers in Canada and the United States to determine the presence of three commonly used agents: cyclophosphamide, ifosfamide, and fluorouracil. Measurable amounts of all three agents were found in 75% of the samples from the pharmacy mixing areas and in 65% of the samples from the administration areas. Clinical studies done with one CSTD, the PhaSeal® system (Carmel Pharma), showed significant reduction in surface contamination in HD compounding areas when the CSTD was used compared to the standard needle-and-syringe technique (Connor et al., 2002; Harrison, Peters, & Bing, 2006; Sessink, Rolf, & Ryden, 1999; Vandenbroucke, 2001).

A number of other CSTD systems, with various methods of capturing HD residue during compounding, have been marketed since 2000. All of the systems are designed to protect the key areas of compounding and administration where studies have identified drug escaping into the environment: vial penetration with needle; leakage from syringe with needle or when removing needle; transfer into an IV solution bag; spiking an IV solution with an IV set; priming the IV set for patient administration; administration of IV push doses; and removal of IV sets from bags, primary sets, or manifolds. Each system offers an access "cap" that locks onto the vial top and provides protection when reconstituting or removing drug from the vial. The cap has a spike or a cannula that penetrates the vial septum and an external, closed device that mates with a specific syringe adapter. This connection between the vial cap and syringe adapter allows needle-safe or needle-free access to the vial. Two of the existing systems use an adapter that contains either covered or recessed spikes allowing transfer of fluid from the syringe and vial. Other systems use a closed male Luer (Luer-Lok™ [Becton, Dickinson and Co.]) instead of a needle-safe adapter that attaches to the syringe. This closed male Luer mates with the specific needle-free adapter on the vial cap opening valves and allows the transfer of fluid between the syringe and vial. Each system has a bag access device that is placed on the IV bag before any drug is added. Each system's bag access device is equipped with the proprietary adapter that allows it to mate with the syringe adapter, either the spiked, needle-safe injector or the needle-free, closed male Luer. The bag adapters allow a closed connection between the drug in the syringe and the IV bag, and a dry connection to the spike of any IV set. Bag adapters allow connecting the IV set and priming the IV line prior to adding drug or, alternatively, to spike at the patient's area using the dry-spike option and back-priming the IV set (usually a secondary set) from the primary (plain) fluid. The closed male Luer connectors are designed to mate with the specific needle-free adapter on IV tubing (Y-sites), creating closed, leak-resistant connections at the patient's line for either IV push administration or additional protection at a tubing-to-tubing connection. The needle-safe systems offer adapters for Y-sites to allow IV push protection and additional tubing protection. The use of these tubing-to-tubing connection devices allows safe removal of either the syringe or secondary tubing from the patient's primary IV setup.

To date, only PhaSeal has been studied in the clinical environment. In laboratory studies, two devices showed similar aerosol and particle capturing performance (Nygren, Gustavsson, & Eriksson, 2005). The capturing capacity for vapors was not tested. In another study, the authors determined that a system in which air can pass in and out during preparation cannot physically be regarded as a closed system according to the NIOSH definition (Nygren, Olofsson, & Johannson, 2008). A clarification of the NIOSH definition, however, led these authors to conclude that compounding systems, like the ones they had studied, should all be regarded as meeting the NIOSH CSTD definition if they are shown to perform according to the specified performance criteria (Nygren, Olofsson, & Johannson, 2009).

Because the CSTD systems have components that are used in the administration of HD doses as well as in the compounding, these devices reduce the potential exposure of nursing staff during administration. Overall reduction of surface contamination should reduce uptake of HD by all staff assigned to any area where HD doses are compounded or administered. Both NIOSH and USP 797 require that if a CSTD is used for HD compounding of sterile doses, then it must be used within an appropriate PEC (NIOSH, 2004; USP, 2008a); a CSTD is not considered a substitute for a PEC or PPE.

Administrative Controls

Administrative controls form the backbone of any safety program. These establish the awareness of an issue and provide clear direction for reducing exposure. Administrative controls include policies, procedures, scheduling practices, staff education and training, validation of competency, and medical surveillance. The safety program must be well established, and staff performance expectations should be clearly defined.

Organizations should have policies and procedures related to safe handling of HDs. Policies should address all aspects of handling these hazardous materials for the protection of employees, patients, customers, and the environment from exposure.
- Policies must address safe storage, transport, administration, and disposal of HDs.
- All employees handling HDs should be required to wear PPE.
- Policies should prohibit eating, drinking, smoking, chewing gum or tobacco, applying cosmetics, and storing food in areas where HDs are used.
- All employees who handle HDs in any capacity, including compounding, administering, spill control, and waste management, must be trained and the training documented.
- Spills should be managed according to the HD spill policy and procedure.
- Written policies should address medical surveillance of employees involved in the handling of HDs.
- Quality improvement programs should include monitoring of compliance with HD policies and procedures (Ellsworth-Wolk & Maxson, 2005).

The risks of exposure to HDs in the workplace must be made clear to all staff at every level, including aides, housekeepers, and laundry service workers, as well as healthcare professionals. USP 797 emphasizes administrative controls for the safe compounding of HDs by mandating conditions that protect HCWs and other personnel in the preparation and storage areas (USP, 2008a). USP 797, OSHA, and NIOSH require extensive training of all personnel who handle HDs in the safety procedures and equipment necessary to perform the specific task; this includes the PEC, PPE, and any emergency procedures associated with acute exposure or spill control. The effectiveness of training must be verified prior to beginning any work with HDs, and ongoing training must be documented at least annually. Training in work practices also must include the following: aseptic manipulation; negative pressure technique; correct use of safety equipment; containment, cleanup, and disposal procedures for breakages and spills; and treatment of personnel for contact and inhalation exposure. (See the Staff Education and Training section for a full discussion of education and training for HD handlers.)

Administrative controls also should include a medical surveillance program (OSHA, 1995). Medical surveillance involves collecting and interpreting data to detect changes in the health status of working populations potentially exposed to hazardous substances. NIOSH provides direction for establishing such a program in its publication *Workplace Solution: Medical Surveillance for Health Care Workers Exposed to Hazardous Drugs* (NIOSH, 2007). Clear policies should be established for workers regarding reproductive risks and alternative duty, as well as reasonable scheduling patterns to reduce the potential for overexposure. (See the Medical Surveillance of Healthcare Workers Handling Hazardous Drugs section for details about medical surveillance for HD handlers.)

Work Practice Controls

Another way to reduce occupational exposure to HDs is to use appropriate work practices. Work practices must be designed to minimize the generation of HD contamination and maximize the containment of inadvertent contamination that occurs during all routine tasks involving HDs and in the event of a breakage or spill. Work practice controls are an extension of other aspects of the hierarchy of controls. They are similar to administrative controls in that they are the established procedures. Work practices often involve the consistent and appropriate use of engineering controls and PPE to minimize exposure.

A critical examination of the existing work practices is necessary to identify potential opportunities for HD exposure. Certain work practices can result in surface contamination with HDs, such as

- Exiting and reentering a BSC to obtain additional equipment without changing gloves
- Failing to wipe off HD vials/ampoules prior to compounding to remove drug residue
- Inadequate cleaning of spills on equipment, such as infusion pumps
- Priming IV tubing with HDs instead of saline or priming tubing outside the PEC unless a dry-spiked connection and Y-site CSTD are available and used.
- Inadequate hand-washing after HD handling activities
- Contaminating hands and other areas while removing PPE.

Many possible causes of surface contamination exist. Direct observation of nurses', pharmacists', and others' techniques of preparation, handling, and administration may yield information about potential sources of contamination and its spread. If potential sources of surface contamination are not identified, they cannot be eliminated.

The following work practices are likely to result in decreased surface contamination.

- Gather all necessary supplies before placing hands in the PEC.
- Double gloving is recommended by both NIOSH and USP 797, and the gloves must be tested for use with HDs.
- Change gloves every 30 minutes and whenever contamination occurs.
- Remove contaminated gloves carefully, turning them inside out to protect bare hands from coming in contact with the outside of the gloves.
- Wash hands after removing gloves and prior to donning new gloves.
- Place waste generated in compounding (e.g., outer gloves, vials, gauze) in a sealed plastic bag before removing it from the PEC.
- Discard the sealed bag containing used equipment in a puncture-proof HD waste receptacle placed immediately outside the PEC.
- Avoid reaching into sealed bags used to transport drugs without PPE. Visually examine the contents of the sealed bag. If visible leakage is present, do not open the outer bag. To reduce the risk of exposure, verify the dose at the administration site. For example, one RN wearing PPE can remove the drug container from the bag while another nurse performs a double check without touching the drug container. An alternative is to use clear sealable bags for transport so that the doses can be verified without removing the drug containers from the bag. This practice might not be possible if ultraviolet light–blocking bags are used.
- Protect work surfaces where HD containers are set down with a plastic-backed pad.
- Use locking connections on all IV delivery devices.
- Use and dispose of sharps carefully.
- Avoid "unspiking" IV bags or bottles. Discontinue and discard infusion bags and bottles with tubing intact.

- Place HD disposal containers near the workspace.
- Keep the lid closed on HD disposal containers except when placing contaminated materials in them.
- Avoid touching equipment (e.g., infusion pumps, computer keyboards, telephones) when wearing gloves used to handle HD containers.
- Clean countertops and other surfaces in the work area after completion of HD handling.

Personal Protective Equipment

The use of PPE is one of the most effective ways for HCWs to prevent occupational exposure to HDs. Since the widespread use of PPE, employee exposure to HDs has decreased. Studies have demonstrated that gloves provide protection against skin contact with tested HDs, and preventing skin exposure decreases symptoms in people with occupational contact with HDs (Nygren & Lundgren, 1997; Valanis et al., 1993a; Valanis, Vollmer, Labuhn, & Glass, 1993b). ONS defines PPE as chemotherapy-tested gloves, gowns made of materials tested for use with chemotherapy, respirators, and face shields or goggles (Polovich, Whitford, & Olsen, 2009).

Gloves: Designated chemotherapy gloves should be worn during all HD-handling activities. Glove thickness, type, and time worn are major determinants of their permeability by HDs. The American Society for Testing and Materials (ASTM, 2005) has developed a standard for testing gloves against permeability by HDs. Gloves are not tested for all known HDs because of the cost; however, for gloves to be labeled for use with chemotherapy, they must be tested with the following seven drugs from different classifications:
- Carmustine
- Cyclophosphamide
- Doxorubicin
- Etoposide
- Fluorouracil
- Paclitaxel
- Thiotepa.

Two additional HDs can be selected from a list provided by ASTM for permeation testing. All drugs used for testing must be purchased from pharmaceutical drug manufacturers or authorized distributors and prepared using the manufacturer's recommendations.

The test results are reported as the amount of time it takes for the drugs to permeate from the outer surface to the inner surface of the glove. Gloves used in handling HDs should have a minimum permeation time of 30 minutes. The most recent standard is ASTM D6978-05, in which the minimum limit of detection is 0.01 mcg/cm^2/min. The older standard (ASTM F739) from 1999 was not specific to gloves and had a minimum limit of detection of 0.1 mcg/cm^2/min, which is only one-tenth as stringent as the new standard. HDs used in testing gloves often are listed on the glove box along with the permeability results. Alternatively, study results may be found in information provided by glove manufacturers. Gloves not tested for use with HDs should not be used for HD handling because their ability to protect against chemical permeation is unknown.

Powder-free gloves are preferred for HD handling because powder may absorb contaminants, be dispersed, and increase the possibility of surface contamination. OSHA (1995) recommended changing gloves every 60 minutes and immediately if contamination occurs. However, based on permeability testing, the maximum recommended wear time for gloves is 30 minutes, and they should be removed immediately if torn, punctured, or contaminated. Visual inspection of gloves to assess for pinhole leaks is a prudent practice, as variability of glove integrity within lots has been identified.

Double gloving is recommended for all activities involving HDs. The likelihood of permeation through two layers of gloves is small; however, wearing two pairs of gloves helps to protect the HCW's hands from contamination that can occur when removing gloves. The inner glove should be worn under the gown sleeve, and the outer glove should be placed over the gown cuff. This technique ensures that skin on the wrist area is not exposed and facilitates correct sequencing (i.e., outer glove, gown, inner glove) during removal of PPE (ASHP, 2006).

Concerns about latex sensitivity have prompted testing of newer glove materials. In one study, thin-gauge 0.0045-inch nitrile gloves demonstrated efficacy in preventing penetration by 11 antineoplastic drugs (Gross & Groce, 1998). The glove thickness required to provide protection from HD permeation varies with the type of glove material.

Connor and Xiang (2000) studied the effect of isopropyl alcohol on the permeation of gloves exposed to antineoplastic agents. They found that the use of isopropyl alcohol for cleaning and decontaminating did not have a significant impact on the integrity of either latex or nitrile gloves during the limited study period of 30 minutes. This is an important finding, as alcohol is used routinely as a disinfectant in BSCs during HD preparation. Figure 3 presents a summary of recommendations for glove use in HD handling.

Figure 3. Recommendations for Glove Use in Hazardous Drug Handling

- Use gloves that have been tested with hazardous drugs.
- Select powder-free gloves.
- Inspect gloves for visible defects.
- Wear double gloves for all handling activities.
- Change gloves every 30 minutes or immediately if damaged or contaminated.

Gowns: Gowns that provide adequate protection from HDs should be disposable and made of a lint-free, low-permeability fabric. They should have a solid front (back closure) and knit or elastic cuffs (ASHP, 2006; OSHA, 1995). Laboratory coats and other cloth fabrics absorb fluids, so they provide an inadequate barrier to HDs and should not be used. The existing guidelines do not contain a recommendation for the maximum length of time that a gown should be worn. Because no recommendations are stated in the literature, at a minimum, remove and discard the gown immediately if contaminated, at the end of handling activities, or when leaving the drug-handling area.

No standard currently exists for testing gowns for permeability by HDs. However, several gown materials have been found to provide protection. Harrison and Kloos (1999) evaluated the permeability of six commercially available protective gowns by splash-testing them with 15 antineoplastic agents. Gowns with polyethylene or vinyl coatings provided adequate splash protection and prevented penetration of the antineoplastic agents. Unfortunately, they made the researchers feel warmer and were less breathable than the more permeable gowns. Two gowns made of polypropylene were permeable in less than one minute, leading the researchers to recommend that they not be used in HD handling.

The purpose of wearing a gown is to protect the HCW's clothing from HD contamination. Gowns should always be worn during chemotherapy preparation and when administering chemotherapy by any route (ASHP, 2006; OSHA, 1995). Gowns should also be used when disposing of HD containers and when handling patients' HD-contaminated excreta, as splashing and contamination of clothing are possible (OSHA, 1995). This represents a change in practice for many nurses but is necessary to provide adequate protection against exposure to HDs.

Gowns worn while preparing HDs should be removed before leaving the preparation area, before the inner gloves are removed (ASHP, 1990). Gowns worn while administering HDs should be changed when leaving the patient care area or immediately if contaminated. The practice of hanging up a gown between uses may lead to surface contamination and contamination of clothing when reapplied. Gowns are intended for single use and should not be worn more than once.

Eye and facial protection: A plastic face shield should be worn in situations where eye, mouth, or nasal splashing is possible (such as during a bladder instillation of HDs). Goggles protect the eyes, but not the face, against spraying. Surgical masks do not provide respiratory protection and should not be relied upon for protection against aerosolized powders or liquids, such as during drug preparation. For HD preparation, the PEC provides eye and face protection (ASHP, 1990; OSHA, 1995). For HD administration, working below eye level greatly reduces the likelihood of eye and facial splashing.

Areas where HDs are handled should have a sink with an eyewash station. Two functionally equivalent and cost-effective alternatives to an eyewash station are an IV bag of 0.9% sodium chloride solution (normal saline) connected to IV tubing or an irrigation bag of water or normal saline with attached tubing, which can be used to flush the eyes (ASHP, 2006). To protect sterility, tubing should be connected immediately before use.

Respiratory protection: Respiratory protection is necessary when drug aerosols are present, such as when administering aerosolized HDs or when cleaning up spills. A surgical mask is not a respirator and does not protect against aerosols or vapors. For most activities requiring respiratory protection, a fit-tested NIOSH-approved N95 or more protective respirator, such as that worn for tuberculosis protection, is sufficient to protect against airborne particles. These respirators offer no protection against gases and vapors. If gas or vapor exposure is possible, wear an air-purifying respirator that includes both a gas/vapor cartridge in combination with an N95 or greater particulate filter. Check the material safety data sheet (MSDS) for appropriate respiratory protection to use based on the situation (NIOSH, 1996).

Drug Compounding

USP General Chapter 797 identifies the term *compounded sterile preparations* (CSPs) to include all compounded dosage forms that must be sterile when they are administered to patients and manufactured sterile products that are either prepared strictly according to the instructions appearing in manufacturers' approved labeling (product package inserts) or prepared differently than published in such labeling (USP, 2008a).

Compounding includes preparing, mixing, and transferring drug between containers. USP 797 defines the conditions in which sterile compounding should take place to ensure the protection of patients. In the 2008 revision to USP 797, sterile compounding of HDs is also addressed, and compounding conditions have been modified to ensure the protection of HCWs.

Drug compounding represents a significant risk of exposure to HDs because of the potentially contaminated drug vials, the higher concentrations of drugs handled, and the multiple manipulations required. The goal of using engineering controls, PPE, and meticulous work practices is to reduce the opportunities for worker exposure during HD compounding and related activities.

Many groups, including ASHP and ONS, have published updated guidelines for special precautions in all HD-related activities (ASHP, 2006; Polovich et al., 2009). OSHA addressed this worker hazard in the 1980s and 1990s, and NIOSH produced a significant update in its 2004 alert, *Preventing Occupational Exposure to Antineoplastic and Other Hazardous Drugs in Health Care Settings* (NIOSH, 2004; OSHA, 1995). As noted, the

2008 revision of USP 797 addresses compounding sterile doses of HDs (USP, 2008a). USP 797 is an enforceable standard that mandates certain precautions during the storage and compounding of sterile doses of HDs (USP, 2008a). The standards in USP 797 are intended to apply to all individuals who prepare CSPs and all places where CSPs are prepared (e.g., hospitals and other healthcare institutions, patient treatment clinics, pharmacies, physicians' practice facilities, other locations and facilities) and applies to all healthcare personnel who prepare, store, and transport CSPs (USP, 2008a).

General Information

All procedures for compounding HDs, such as reconstituting, mixing, and transferring a drug, must take place in a PEC. A PEC is defined as a device that provides an ISO Class 5 environment for the exposure of critical sites when compounding any sterile preparation (USP, 2008a). Critical sites include any location where component or fluid pathway surfaces (e.g., vial septa or injection ports) or openings (e.g., opened ampoules, needle hubs) are exposed and are at risk of direct contact with air, moisture (e.g., oral and mucosal secretions), or touch contamination (USP, 2008a). For compounding sterile doses of HDs, the appropriate PECs include BSCs and CACIs (ASHP, 2006; NIOSH, 2004; USP, 2008a). These devices protect the environment and the operator from HD residue and provide the needed "clean" (i.e., ISO Class 5) environment for sterile compounding. An extensive discussion of engineering controls may be found in the Hierarchy of Controls section.

It must be accepted that PECs do not eliminate the *generation* of contamination during HD compounding and may not be entirely effective in containing HD aerosols and residue. Secondary controls, such as PPE and stringent work practices, are required to maximize the usefulness of all PECs. Worker training on the correct techniques in using the PEC and other safety devices is critical in establishing an effective safe handling program.

NIOSH and USP 797 agree that HD storage and compounding should be separated from other drug activities with environments that have adequate ventilation, ACPH, and environments that are at negative pressure to surrounding areas. These engineering requirements help to contain any contamination generated in the storage or compounding of HDs and limit its spread out of the immediate work area (NIOSH, 2004; USP, 2008a). Discussions of buffer areas and ante areas may be found in Hierarchy of Controls.

Primary Engineering Control Work Practices

The Class II BSC and the CACI require somewhat different techniques for accessing and operating the PECs for compounding HDs. The CACI has attached sleeves and gloves that limit the movement of the operator and require that all drugs, supplies, and completed doses be placed into and removed from the cabinet through transfer chambers, also known as *pass-throughs*. Training and practice are standard requirements for the use of all equipment.

Cleaning and disinfecting the PEC is required prior to beginning sterile compounding. To remove HD residue, a surface decontamination is required (see Table 5). Disinfectants, especially alcohol, do not deactivate HDs (Dorr, 2001). While nothing has been shown to deactivate all HDs, many of the HD MSDSs recommend sodium hypochlorite (bleach) solution as an appropriate deactivating agent (Johnson & Janosik, 1989). Researchers have shown that strong oxidizing agents, such as sodium hypochlorite, are effective deactivators of many HDs (Benvenuto et al., 1993; Hansel et al., 1997). Sodium hypochlorite with a detergent and neutralizer

Table 5. Bugs Versus Drugs: What Are Decontamination and Cleaning?

Cleaning and *surface decontamination* are very general terms that signify the removal of contamination. In sterile compounding of hazardous drugs (HDs), contamination may take the form of viable organisms (*bugs*) or HD residue (*drugs*). **Disinfection** neutralizes viable organisms; **deactivation** neutralizes chemical residue. No one agent has been found that does both reliably and consistently. Residue left on compounding surfaces from either disinfection or deactivation must be removed by physically wiping with appropriate wipers and rinsing agents (a no-residue cleaner or sterile water for irrigation).

Desired Effect	Considerations and Concerns	Possible Agents
Disinfection—removal of viable organism (bugs) Disinfectants are classified as low, intermediate, and high level based on which organism they kill and the concentration and contact time required.	Disinfectants are used to remove viable organisms from surfaces in the compounding area and to sanitize gloves during sterile compounding. Disinfectants may be hampered by the presence of blood or other biologic fluids or other residue that requires removal ("cleaning") prior to or in conjunction with disinfection. Certain disinfectants incorporate a detergent into the solution. Low- or no-residue disinfectants are preferred to avoid rinsing. Controlled Environment Testing Association (2007) and USP 1072 (U.S. Pharmacopeia, 2008b) provide information on different levels of disinfectants and sterilants that are useful against a variety of organisms and may be used in rotation with sterile isopropyl alcohol to improve surface decontamination.	***Disinfectants*** Intermediate level • Sterile 70% isopropyl alcohol • Iodophor • Phenolic • Accelerated hydrogen peroxide (efficacy based on concentration plus contact time) High level • Chlorine (efficacy based on concentration plus contact time)
Sanitizing Sterile gloves are easily contaminated (bugs and drugs) and should be sanitized with a disinfectant as needed during compounding.	Hand or glove sanitizers should be available in the sterile compounding area. With HD compounding, gloves are also contaminated with HD residue. DO NOT handle sanitizers with dirty gloves. Use wipers to touch bottles. NEVER spray the sanitizer onto the gloves (or other surfaces), as this will transfer the HD residue. Spray or place gel on the wiper and wipe off (sanitize) the gloves. Contain and discard all wipers used on potentially HD-contaminated surfaces as HD waste.	***Hand/Glove Sanitizers*** • Alcohol-based gels • Disinfectant gel • 70% sterile isopropyl alcohol spray
Deactivation (drugs) Removes chemical residue by degradation or inactivation. Some HDs are potent chemicals with resistance to deactivation.	Deactivating agents may be strong chemicals that present their own problems in clinical use. No one agent has been shown to inactivate or neutralize all HDs. Some chemicals are effective against some HDs. Some HDs, however, degrade to mutagenic by-products upon treatment with some chemicals. Residue from deactivation must still be removed from the affected surfaces.	***Deactivating agents*** • Material safety data sheets (MSDSs) list agents to use in response to a spill. Many list **sodium hypochlorite (bleach)** as effective. Concentration and contact time must be considered. • Package inserts for HDs list some agents that degrade HDs. **Sodium thiosulfate** deactivates certain HDs. Mechlorethamine, for example, is neutralized with 5% sodium thiosulfate and 5% sodium bicarbonate solution for 45 minutes.
Surface decontamination (drug and other residue) Removes contamination (residue) from a nondisposable surface to a disposable one using detergent and good wipers followed by rinsing.	Low-sudsing and low-residue detergents may be used to remove contamination from surfaces in the primary engineering control (PEC) or adjacent surfaces (counters, storage bins, floors, etc.). All cleaning must be done wearing double gloves, and all disposable wipers, towels, gauze pads, etc. must be contained in sealable plastic bags and then discarded as hazardous waste. Surface decontamination must be followed by rinsing. Disinfect all PEC surfaces prior to compounding. The amount of HD contamination placed into the BSC or isolator may be reduced by surface decontamination (i.e., wiping down) of HD vials. Although no wipe-down procedures have been studied, the use of gauze moistened with alcohol, sterile water, peroxide, or sodium hypochlorite solutions may be effective.	***Detergents*** • High pH soap-type cleaners are recommended in the MSDS and other literature. • Dilute all cleaners according to manufacturer instructions. • Prepare cleaners and disinfectants carefully. • Use only freshly prepared cleaners and disinfectants.

Note. Based on information from American Society of Health-System Pharmacists, 2006; Benvenuto et al., 1993; Controlled Environment Testing Association, 2007; Hansel et al., 1997; Johnson & Janosik, 1989; U.S. Pharmacopeia, 2008b.

is commercially available as Surface Safe®* (Hospira, Inc.) and has been used to decontaminate PECs. The oxidizing bleach solution is combined with a detergent on a pad (fabric wipe) that provides physical cleaning action along with some deactivation. The neutralizer protects stainless steel surfaces and also deactivates certain HDs that are not affected by bleach. Decontamination is recommended at least daily for a PEC that runs 24 hours per day but is used only for one shift; a PEC that is used throughout the 24 hours must be decontaminated two to three times daily (ASHP, 2006). Decontamination must be done if a spill has occurred or if visible residue is generated during compounding. Disinfection of the PEC with sterile 70% isopropyl alcohol must be done prior to any sterile compounding and every 30 minutes during continuous compounding (USP, 2008a). Apply spray to the wipes, not the PEC surface, whenever HD compounding has taken place in a PEC to avoid spreading the HD residue. All wipes used to decontaminate or disinfect a PEC used for HDs must be contained and discarded as HD waste.

Universally, good organization will improve compounding regardless of the type of PEC. Select and assemble drugs and all supplies and solutions prior to accessing the PEC. With a BSC, this reduces the need to enter and exit the cabinet, which may cause HD contamination to migrate from the cabinet to the surrounding work area. As the closed CACI does not allow quick access to the work area, lack of organization results in extended compounding time.

USP 797 requires that drugs and supplies brought into the PEC be wiped down or sprayed with sterile 70% isopropyl alcohol to reduce the particulate load and related microbial contamination (USP, 2008a). HD drug vials have been shown to be contaminated with drug residue when they are received from the manufacturer or distributor (Connor, 2005). Removing this contamination is necessary to avoid placing HD residue into the isolator or BSC work area and then transferring it to other surfaces. Although wiping techniques and solutions have not been studied to document what procedure is best, general principles may be applied: use low-linting wipes that meet the intent of USP 797 for sterile compounding; use fresh wipes and discard as HD-contaminated waste; do not reuse wipes; spray the wipe, not the drug vial, to avoid transfer of the HD residue into the air or onto other surfaces; and use fresh gloves for wiping, and change gloves before compounding to avoid transfer of HD residue from the glove surfaces. While Surface Safe* is appropriate for decontaminating the PEC, it may damage the label if applied directly to the drug vial, creating a safety issue for patients if the drug and dose are not visible. Sterile 70% isopropyl alcohol and sterile water for irrigation do not damage the vial label and should be adequate, if used as previously described, in reducing the HD residue.

Only those items needed for immediate compounding should be placed in the work area of the BSC or the main chamber of the CACI. Overcrowding should be avoided inside the PEC as excess supplies can block the airflow, which may breach the containment properties of the Class II BSC. This may also interfere with the HEPA-filtered, unidirectional air in either the BSC or CACI, compromising sterile compounding (ASHP, 1990, 2006; USP, 2008a). Excess supplies in the BSC or main chamber of the CACI may become contaminated from HD residue generated during the compounding process (Sessink et al., 1992). This contamination may then be transferred out of the PEC. Place only those items necessary for drug preparation, a small disposable sharps container, and a heavy-duty zipper-lock bag (for disposal of syringes, vials, and gloves) in the BSC before beginning work. The CACI may be equipped with waste outlets that allow waste to be discarded directly from the main chamber. Containing waste in small zipper-lock bags before placing in HD waste containers provides more robust containment. Items not needed immediately may be left in the transfer chamber of the CACI and accessed as needed. Care must be taken to avoid HD transfer from dirty gloves.

*See Clinical Update on page viii.

The practice of covering the working surface of the PEC with a plastic-backed, absorbent, disposable drape is problematic for both sterile compounding and HD containment. The drape can negatively affect the containment airflow of the BSC (Minoia et al., 1998) and possibly the clean airflow in a CACI with unidirectional air. In-house testing by one manufacturer concluded that the use of a Chemoplus™ Prep Mat (Kendall/Covidien) on the work surface of a Class II BSC does not harm the containment performance as long as the mat remains on the work surface and never blocks the front or rear work zone grills (NuAire, Inc., 2005). USP 797 is currently silent on the addition of a nonsterile mat into the PEC. If used, the mat must be considered contaminated with HD residue. It must be handled carefully, changed routinely (no current recommendations for frequency of changing exist), and discarded as HD waste.

Studies have shown that gloves are routinely contaminated with HD residue during compounding, and transfer of this contamination to other surfaces is common (Sessink et al., 1992). USP 797 requires frequent sanitization of gloves during sterile compounding. While this is also needed with HD compounding, care must be taken not to handle spray bottles with contaminated gloves. Use wipes to act as a barrier between dirty gloves and other surfaces; spray the wipes, not the gloves, with disinfectant; and wipe the gloves and discard the wipes as HD waste. Wearing two pairs of gloves during compounding allows the outer pair to be changed as needed while reducing the exposure to the worker because the inner pair remains intact. In addition, good work practices for all sterile products, as well as HD doses, require frequent hand-washing prior to donning gloves. Hands must be washed with soap and water after removing gloves.

Limitations Specific to the Class II Biologic Safety Cabinet

The effectiveness of the Class II BSC in protecting HCWs and the environment is related to the airflow. Although the cabinet is designed to direct airflow and potential drug contamination away from the worker, this is a very technique-dependent process. Workers should avoid moving their hands in and out of the cabinet during compounding because a disturbance in the airflow may result in directing drug aerosols outside the cabinet. This should be kept in mind whenever there is the possibility of releasing drugs into the environment, such as when an HD container is open and during all drug-transferring activities.

Personal Protective Equipment in Primary Engineering Controls

The use of a Class II BSC does not eliminate the need for PPE, and no studies have documented that a CACI reduces the transfer of HD contamination to the operator during the loading and unloading process. Because spills are possible during any HD handling, PPE must be used to prevent worker exposure. Gowns made of materials that protect from HD permeation and double gloves, tested to the ASTM standard (ASTM, 2005), are universally recommended for HD handling (ASHP, 2006; NIOSH, 2004; OSHA, 1995; Polovich et al., 2009; USP, 2008a). USP 797 requires extensive garbing (gown, gloves, mask, hair and shoe covers) to reduce the transfer of microbial-laden particulates from the worker to the environment and sterile product (USP, 2008a). USP 797 requires two pairs of gloves, the outer one sterile, for compounding sterile preparations (USP, 2008a). When wearing double gloves, tuck the cuff of the inner glove under the gown sleeve and the cuff of the outer glove over the gown sleeve. Change the outer gloves immediately whenever contamination is suspected. Change both gloves if the outer glove is torn, punctured, or contaminated by an obvious spill. At the completion of each batch, the outer gloves should be removed and sealed in a zipper-lock bag. Remove and discard the gown before removing the inner pair of gloves.

Compounding of Sterile Hazardous Drug Doses

Aseptic technique is required for compounding all parenteral drugs to maintain the sterility. CSPs are addressed in USP 797 along with specific training and methods to document competency of aseptic technique (USP, 2008a). Appropriate actions to provide safe CSPs for patients are assumed and will not be addressed here. Meticulous aseptic technique for compounding HDs in ampoules and vials has been described in the literature (Wilson & Solimando, 1981).

Luer-locking syringes and access devices (needles, needleless devices, etc.) must always be used in HD compounding to prevent inadvertent separation of the devices and resulting leakage. Syringes should never be more than three-fourths full when containing the HD dose to prevent separation of the plunger from the syringe barrel during compounding or transport (ASHP, 1990, 2006; OSHA, 1995).

HDs supplied in ampoules (e.g., arsenic trioxide, alemtuzumab, tacrolimus) require special precautions both to prevent microbial contamination and to avoid drug leakage from this open system. When opening ampoules, tap down any drug from the top of the ampoule and wrap a sterile gauze pad around the neck. Break the ampoule carefully using a single sharp motion, aiming the ampoule into a corner of the PEC away from the HEPA filter; do not aim at the operator or open front of the BSC. The gauze will reduce the risk of injury from the sharp edges of the glass, as well as drug contamination from spilling. A filtering device must be used to prevent glass particles from being drawn into the syringe. Using a filtering straw reduces the risk of needlestick associated with withdrawing the drug with a filter needle. The straw, however, has no cover, so care must be taken to keep the packaging for removal and disposal of the straw into a sealed containment bag.

Most HDs are supplied in vials, and some may require reconstitution. When adding liquid to an HD drug vial or withdrawing HD doses from vials, use caution to avoid pressure buildup inside the vial that can result in aerosolization or leakage. Needleless dispensing devices with hydrophobic filters often are used to equilibrate any pressure in the vial, but no evidence is available to support their effectiveness in reducing HD exposure. No filter will prevent the escape of vapors. These devices are not closed systems and may have open channels into the drug vial. In general, these devices do not lock onto the vial and may dislodge during use, resulting in large spills. These devices, if used, should be attached to one vial only and discarded with the empty vial into a containment disposal bag.

Negative Pressure Technique

When adding diluent to a vial or withdrawing liquid from a vial, use the negative pressure technique described by Wilson and Solimando (1981). Whether the syringe contains air or liquid, do NOT push on the plunger when the needle is in the vial. Use a syringe that is large enough to manipulate excess air, and after making the initial puncture with the needle, pull BACK on the plunger, drawing air into the syringe and creating negative pressure in the vial. This "vacuum" will draw the liquid into the vial without pushing the plunger and pressurizing the HD vial. Repeat the process until the diluent is transferred to the vial and the air is in the syringe. If possible, keep the needle in the vial while swirling to reconstitute the HD. If the volume of the dose may be removed from the vial without removing the needle or correcting the air volume, do so, as a second puncture in the vial septum presents an opportunity for leakage. If the needle must be removed from the vial, place the vial upright on the work surface and move the needle into the air space above the drug. Withdraw just enough air into the syringe so that there is a pull on the plunger, demonstrating the negative pressure in the vial. Hold on to the vial and plunger, and remove the needle from the vial septum. This technique should avoid generating positive pressure or leaking drug around the needle or access device.

When withdrawing liquid from a vial, draw up slightly less air into the syringe than the volume of the dose to be withdrawn. After the initial puncture, draw back on the plunger, creating negative pressure in the HD vial. Invert the vial to allow liquid to enter the syringe, repeating the process until the correct dose is transferred to the syringe. Once the dose volume has been transferred to the syringe, hold the syringe plunger firmly, and place the vial upright on the work surface. Move the needle into the air space above the drug and draw back slightly on the plunger, bringing air into the syringe JUST to the top of the syringe hub, not into the syringe. This clears the HD liquid from the needle. Hold the plunger firmly, as the vacuum in the vial will strain to equilibrate the pressure. Remove the needle from the vial septum. Transfer the dose into an appropriate IV delivery system. Do not recap HD-contaminated needles unless the needle must be removed. If the dose is to be delivered in the syringe, use a one-handed technique to recap the needle to avoid a needlestick. Remove the needle and cap and replace with a syringe cap for transport. Do not transport drug-filled syringes with needles attached.

Wipe down the outside of the drug container (bag or syringe) with moist gauze. Wipe entry ports with alcohol and apply a closure—either a hard plastic or foil seal is appropriate—to prevent any leakage from the port. Seal the drug syringe or container with the attached tubing in a plastic zipper-lock bag that will contain any spilled drug if the container leaks.

Closed-System Drug Transfer Devices

Connor et al. (2002) demonstrated the potential for leakage in compounding HDs using a needle and syringe, as well as leakage in administration when attaching IV sets and priming lines. CSTDs are designed to protect the sites shown to be prone to leakage during HD compounding and administration activities. Unlike PECs, CSTDs actually reduce the generation of HD contamination in the compounding process. CSTDs, as with all safety equipment, require training for proper use and are not 100% effective. Closed systems are currently not available for use with ampoules. See Hierarchy of Controls for additional CSTD discussion.

Spiking IV Bags and Priming Lines

There is a risk of releasing drugs into the environment when spiking IV bags containing HD doses and when priming IV tubing with drug solution into an HD waste container or gauze pad. Vandenbroucke (2001) reported a 25% rate of leakage during the connection of tubing to an infusion bag. A risk of leakage also exists during the connection of the tubing to the patient side of the IV tubing when the tubing is primed with drug-containing solution. The practice of spiking the IV bag and priming the tubing in the PEC prior to adding the HD is one way to avoid this exposure. As studies have shown, the PEC work surface is laden with HD residue (Connor et al., 1999; Sessink et al., 1992). This practice could transfer contamination to the outside of the tubing, resulting in another opportunity for exposure. Priming in the PEC requires communication between the person compounding the drug and the person administering the drug so that the appropriate administration set is selected. Practice settings that use multiple IV pumps and controllers might find this problematic. Some institutions have elected to attach a secondary set to all IV bags or bottles that contain HDs to avoid this issue. Secondary sets are compatible with most IV tubing with a proximal port and a needleless connector. Once spiked, the secondary set may be primed in the PEC or at the bedside using backflow priming from the primary IV solution.

As an alternative, a CSTD component may be used that spikes into the IV bag in the PEC. This infusion adapter provides a dry-spike connection that may be accessed at the patient bedside with a secondary or primary set and eliminates the risks associated with spiking. This device is ideal for backflow priming at the bedside. When priming the line in the PEC, another alternative is to use the closed male Luer connection available with the CSTD systems to lock off the distal end of the IV tubing (usually a secondary set). This provides a closed system for connecting the IV to the needleless Y-site and then allows the secondary set to be removed when the infusion is completed. Removing standard IV sets from the patient's IV setup is known to be a significant source of exposure because drug remains in the tubing. A closed male Luer prevents any leakage on disconnection, thus allowing the dose and tubing to be discarded into a containment bag as needed rather than waiting until the entire setup may be discarded. This system is especially useful when administering an HD regimen that requires multiple IV bags of HDs for a course of therapy. See Hierarchy of Controls for additional CSTD discussion.

Oral Drugs

Compounding of nonsterile doses of HDs (e.g., crushing or breaking oral HD doses to be made into liquids or ointments) or other activities where containment ventilation is desired (such as opening damaged HD containers, etc.) may be done in a non–ISO Class 5, ventilated environment, such as a fume hood (Class I BSC). If nonsterile activities are done in the ISO Class 5 PEC, full decontamination for HD residue and cleaning and disinfection for particulates and biologics are required prior to resuming sterile compounding.

Unit-dose packaging is the preferred method of providing oral HDs; however, not all HDs are available in that form. Although the active drug is contained in the core of some tablets with the tablet surrounded by inactive substances, it is difficult to ascertain which products are manufactured in that manner. Powder from tablets or damaged capsules represents an exposure risk. Any handling of tablets or capsules should be done wearing double gloves with the assumption that exposure is possible (ASHP, 1990, 2006; NIOSH, 2004; OSHA, 1995).

Crushing tablets or opening capsules for administration through feeding tubes is an inappropriate practice. Liquid formulations should be used. Compounding should take place using some type of engineering control to avoid the risk of inhalation of HD powder. If the only control is the PEC for compounding sterile doses, then complete decontamination and disinfection are required prior to its use for sterile products. For nonsterile HD compounding, a gown made of material that protects against HD permeation and double gloves tested to the ASTM (2005) standard are required. Drugs should be delivered in the final dose and form for administration whenever possible to minimize exposure risk.

Safety Measures

All HD doses must be labeled for proper identification. A label on the drug container itself and on the outside of the bag used for transport will alert the handler that special precautions are required (ASHP, 1990, 2006; NIOSH, 2004; OSHA,

1995). Attach a warning label stating, for example, "CAUTION: HAZARDOUS DRUG. HANDLE WITH GLOVES. DISPOSE OF PROPERLY."

All items used in the compounding of HDs are considered contaminated and should be discarded in a hazardous waste container. Discard needles and other sharps in the small sharps container inside the PEC or through waste ports, if applicable. Discard empty vials, used syringes, drapes, and other items used in drug compounding in the zipper-lock bag. Remove the outer gloves and place them in a zipper-lock bag. Decontaminate any containers stored in the PEC (sharps container, etc.) with bleach or another solution before removing them from the PEC, and place them into the lined hazardous waste container. Carefully remove the gown and then the inner gloves to avoid contaminating skin and clothing. Contain all PPE in zipper-lock bags and discard in the hazardous waste container. Seal the HD waste container if any waste is placed in it that is not contained in a secondary bag. Wash hands with soap and water before leaving the preparation area. Gloves and gowns should not be worn outside the drug preparation area.

Drug Administration

HDs can be administered by a variety of delivery systems and routes in which drugs are directed systemically, regionally, or locally. Although most HDs are given intravenously, alternative routes of administration are sometimes used. Many drugs are administered intra-arterially, by subcutaneous or intramuscular injection, orally, topically, by inhalation, and into bodily cavities. As new treatments become available, alternative routes and delivery systems are likely to be more common. Several drug delivery systems are being studied for their future application in HD administration. These delivery systems include intraosseous vascular access, convection-enhanced delivery, and nanoparticle-polymer drug delivery systems (Muehlbauer et al., 2006; Muthu & Singh, 2009). When therapies include HDs, safe handling precautions are necessary to protect HCWs from exposure.

HDs may be administered in nontraditional settings, such as surgical and procedural suites and interventional and radiology procedural rooms. HDs also are administered for nonmalignant populations and in nonmalignant settings (see Figure 4). Guidelines for HD preparation, administration, disposal, excreta management, aftercare, and PPE apply for all routes and in all settings because giving HDs by any route involves an inherent opportunity for exposure. Recommendations for preventing exposure have evolved over the years as new information has become available. Guidelines established by ASHP (1990) and OSHA (1995) were based on studies of workplace contamination during preparation and administration. Updated versions of these pioneering guidelines have since been published (ASHP, 2006; NIOSH, 2004).

Figure 4. Nonmalignant Conditions Treated With Hazardous Drugs

- Actinic keratosis
- Alzheimer disease: Clinical trials
- Autoimmune inner ear disease
- Autoimmune neurologic disorders
  - Multiple sclerosis
  - Guillain-Barré syndrome
  - Neuromyelitis optica
- Chronic active hepatitis
- Chronic autoimmune neuropathies
  - Anti-myelin–associated glycoprotein (IgM-MAG) neuropathies
  - Chronic inflammatory demyelinating neuropathy
  - Multifocal motor neuropathy
- Crohn disease
- Glomerulonephritis
- Idiopathic nephritic syndrome
- Inflammatory bowel disease
- Inflammatory myopathies
  - Polymyositis
  - Dermatomyositis, body myositis
- Juvenile dermatomyositis
- Juvenile idiopathic arthritis
- Mixed connective tissue disease
- Neuromuscular disease
  - Duchene dystrophy
- Paraneoplastic neurologic disorders
- Parkinson disease: Clinical trials
- Psoriasis, psoriatic arthritis
- Pulmonary diseases
  - Cystic fibrosis
  - Idiopathic pulmonary fibrosis
- Status post–organ transplantation
- Sarcoidosis
- Scleroderma
- Sickle-cell disease
- Sjögren syndrome
- Stiff-person syndrome
- Systemic lupus erythematosus
- Trophoblastic disease
- Vasculitis
  - Behçet disease
  - Microscopic polyangiopathy
  - Polyarteritis, polyarteritis nodosa
  - Primary cerebral vasculitis
  - Wegener granulomatosis

Note. Based on information from Bertsias et al., 2008, 2010; Brogan & Dillon, 2000; Connor & McDiarmid, 2006; Dalakas, 2008, 2010a, 2010b; Dayton, 1996; Fox, 2000; Gulati et al., 2001; Guthrie et al., 2007; Harris et al., 2003; Kendall et al., 2003; Lasak et al., 2001; National Cancer Institute, 2008; Parra, 2000; Smolen et al., 2007; Srinivasan & Slomovic, 2007; Visco et al., 2009.

Figure 5. General Recommendations for Administration of Hazardous Drugs (HDs)

- Ensure appropriate supplies for administration are available.
- Have access to a spill kit.
- Wash hands thoroughly before donning personal protective equipment (PPE).
- Wear two pairs of chemotherapy-tested gloves (National Institute for Occupational Safety and Health [NIOSH], 2004).
- Wear a face shield if there is a chance of the HD splashing.
- Wear a NIOSH-approved respirator if HD aerosols may be present.
- Inspect the drug delivery bag and its contents prior to handling.
- Don PPE before reaching into the delivery bag to remove the drug container.
- Remove gloves and gown in such a way as to prevent transfer of HD contamination to the skin.
- Whenever possible, avoid touching equipment with gloved hands after handling HDs.
- Do not hang up gowns and reuse them.
- Wash hands with soap and water (as opposed to alcohol-based hand gels) because friction and rinsing are necessary to assist in removing HD contamination.
- Perform all work below eye level.
- Use a closed-system drug transfer device when available.

Many HD safe handling precautions are similar no matter what route of administration is used or the location. Those precautions that apply in all situations are listed in Figure 5 (ASHP, 2006; OSHA, 1995; Polovich et al., 2009).

The following sections detail safe handling recommendations for specific routes of HD administration.

Intravenous Infusions

Whenever possible, IV bags containing HDs should be spiked in a PEC to prevent contamination due to inadvertent puncturing of the bag (ASHP, 2006). If spiking at the administration location is unavoidable, it should be done below eye level and the tubing back-primed with nondrug solution. Some manufacturers of CSTDs also offer a "dry spike" adapter, which fits between the IV bag and the IV tubing spike. The adapter prevents HCWs from inadvertently spiking through the side of the IV bag, prevents splashing of HDs, and also allows for backflushing of neutral solution using closed-system components. Under no circumstances should tubing be primed in such a way as to allow the escape of HDs into the environment (e.g., priming into gauze pads, sinks, or trash containers).

Locking connections (e.g., Luer) should be used to securely attach all IV tubings. A CSTD attached to IV tubing can prevent leakage and may prevent aerosolization that may occur because of inadvertent disconnection or at completion of the infusion (ASHP, 2006).

Current ASHP and NIOSH guidelines strongly discourage unspiking HD bags at the end of an infusion and recommend using new tubing with each dose of chemotherapy. Changing the bag and tubing together helps to prevent potential contamination associated with unspiking. Whenever possible, a nondrug solution should be used to flush tubing prior to disconnecting. This can be accomplished by infusing HDs through a secondary IV tubing which, when empty, is flushed by back-priming with the primary solution. A CSTD attached to the end of the IV tubing will prevent leakage during disconnection. When disconnecting a chemotherapy infusion without a CSTD, an absorbent pad should be placed beneath the connection and/or the connection wrapped with gauze to contain droplets (Polovich et al., 2009).

Dispose of PPE and other potentially contaminated items by sealing them in a plastic bag and discarding them in an HD disposal container. Alternatively, items can be placed directly into a hard-sided container specifically designated for HD waste (ASHP, 1990). At the conclusion of the infusion, wash hands and don appropriate PPE. Remove the bag or bottle containing the HD with the tubing attached. Discard all contaminated material as previously described, and wash hands with soap and water.

Intravenous Injections

Place a plastic-backed absorbent pad under the patient's arm to absorb leaks and prevent HD contact with the patient's skin during IV injections (ASHP, 2006; NIOSH, 2004). Although needleless systems reduce the chance of needlesticks, they do not prevent leaks at connection points. A CSTD can help to prevent leakage and possible aerosolization associated with connecting and disconnecting a syringe. If a CSTD is not used, wrap sterile gauze around injection ports during IV injections to reduce the potential for environmental contamination when attaching or removing the syringe (ASHP, 2006; NIOSH, 2004). Dispose of all contaminated materials as previously described.

Intramuscular or Subcutaneous Injections

For intramuscular or subcutaneous injections of HDs, use syringes with locking connections that are less than three-fourths full. Place an absorbent pad on the work area while connecting the needle to the syringe. Do not expel air from the syringe or prime the needle. After administering the drug, do NOT recap, clip, or crush the needle. Place the syringe with the attached needle directly into a puncture-proof container specifically designed for HD waste (ASHP, 2006; NIOSH, 2004). Remove and dispose of PPE.

Oral Agents

Because of the chance of inhalation exposure, manipulation of oral forms, such as breaking, crushing, or mixing tablets with food or fluids, should not be performed outside of a PEC. Even intact HD tablets or capsules may be coated with residual HD dust (ASHP, 2006). In addition to gloves, PPE should include a gown and face shield if there is a potential for sprays, aerosols, or splattering of the agent, such as with liquid HDs. For unit-dose packages, open carefully so as not to touch the tablets or capsules. Place HDs directly into a medicine cup. Protect the work area with a plastic-backed absorbent pad if necessary.

Nasal Enteral Tube and Enterostomy Tube Delivery

A nasogastric/nasoenteric tube is used when patients require short-term enteral nutrition. The tip of the tube is located in the fundus of the stomach. For patients who are at high risk for aspiration, the tip may be advanced into the jejunum. An enterostomy tube is used for long-term enteral nutrition or decompression, with the tip placed in the stomach or jejunum. Placement of the tube may affect absorption of medications. See Figure 6 for HD preparation and administration via nasogastric or enterostomy tubes.

Because of an increase in the number of U.S. Food and Drug Administration–approved oral HDs (Weingart et al., 2008), enteral tubes have become more common for the delivery of HDs. Research is limited on the use of nasoenteric and enterostomy tubes for HD administration and professional education and role responsibilities (e.g., RN and pharmacist) related to this procedure (Cantarini, McFarquhar, Smith, Bailey, & Marshall, 2004). However, a plethora of literature exists related to oral and nonhazardous medication administration by that method. This administration modality represents an opportunity for HD exposure (Bankhead et al., 2009; Connor & Eisenberg, 2010; Williams, 2008).

Figure 6. Hazardous Drug Preparation and Administration Via Nasogastric or Enterostomy Tubes

1. Identify the type of tube and tip placement.
2. Identify the type of enteral feeding, if present.
3. Discuss the first two considerations with the pharmacy and medical team, as they may affect drug dosing and dilution variables for pharmacy reconstitution. It will also be necessary to determine when feedings can be resumed to prevent alteration of drug bioavailability.
4. The American Society for Parenteral and Enteral Nutrition does not recommend adding medication directly to enteral feedings. The drug package inserts and other drug text may recommend taking the unaltered medication with food. This will need to be discussed with the medical and pharmacy team. Drug-drug and drug-food considerations must also be discussed with the physician and pharmacist/nutritional team.
5. If the enteral tubing system has more than one lumen, administer the medication separately through the nonenteral lumen.
6. Equipment preparation: Adapt the Washburn setup.
   a. Absorbent pad to place under tube-syringe connection
   b. Closed-system drug transfer device
   c. Personal protective equipment and mask
   d. Syringe and sterile saline for flushing before, between medications, and after
   e. Hazardous drug disposal container
7. When capsules and tablets are crushed, mix with sterile water.
8. Stop the feeding and flush the tube with at least 15 ml of sterile water.
9. Reconstituted suspensions or solutions are to be administered in a 30 ml syringe.
10. Flush the tube lumen between medications. CAUTION: Consider the patient's volume status.
11. Following completion of all the medication, administer a final flush of 15 ml of sterile water before capping the tube lumen or resuming enteral administration.
12. The feedings may be delayed for 30 minutes or longer when appropriate to avoid altering the bioavailability of the drug.

Note. Based on information from Bankhead et al., 2009.

Solid oral forms must be crushed to allow administration by tube. Current HD safe handling recommendations do not recommend crushing oral HDs outside of an engineering control. Not all medications are suitable for crushing. Dosage forms that should not be crushed include sustained-release/extended-release/slow-release tablets, enteric-coated tablets, film-coated tablets, and buccal/sublingual forms (Kaufman, 2009; Mitchell, 2010; Williams, 2008) (see Table 6). An up-to-date list of medications that should not be crushed, including many HDs, can be found at www.ismp.org/Tools/DoNotCrush.pdf (Mitchell, 2010). Nurses should consult the manufacturer's prescribing information for recommendations for specific drugs.

Ideally, HD solutions and suspensions are prepared within a designated engineering control and provided in an oral syringe for administration by tube. The use of parenteral syringes with Luer-lock connections may increase the chance of misadministration by the IV route. To facilitate a closed system, modify the Washburn (2007) bladder instillation setup, using a closed-system connector with a Foley tip adapter. Attach the syringe or infusion bag to the connector-adapter setup. Then, attach to the female opening of the nasogastric tube/enterostomy tube system (see Figure 7).

Some drug references suggest that tablets may be dispersed in water or apple juice, stirred until dissolved, and then administered by tube (Turkoski, Lance, & Tomsik, 2009).

Topical Agents

Cream or gel formulations of HDs are applied directly to the skin and are absorbed into cancerous lesions. The indications for topical HDs include squamous cell carcinoma and basal cell carcinoma (NCI, 1998), cutaneous T-cell lymphoma (Mallick, 2007; NCI, 1998), penile cancer (American Cancer Society, 2009), and some non-oncology indications. Although little information exists concerning safety practices for topical HDs, dermal absorption is a primary concern for HCWs (Kromhout et al., 2000; NIOSH, 2004). Therefore, the same precautions used for oral agents should be followed. Clothes and linens that come in contact with the topical HD should be handled with PPE. For isolated lesions, cover with gauze to prevent linen and clothing contamination. Keep the HD container in a zipper-lock bag, separate from all other medications, and handle only with PPE.

Intracavitary Administration

Intracavitary administration includes the instillation of HDs into the bladder, peritoneum, chest, or other body cavity. These procedures represent a significant opportunity for exposure because the drug delivery equipment used is not designed to protect HCWs. Washburn (2007) described a closed administration system for use with any type of catheter that has a female opening (e.g., Foley catheter, feeding tube, suprapubic catheter, chest tube) by combining several pieces of equipment. A food-dye test demonstrated that leakage did not occur when using this system. Figure 7 shows the Washburn setup.

For intracavitary HD administration, select equipment with a closed system or locking connections whenever possible. Wear PPE, including a face shield if locking connections are not available because of the chance of splashing. Place plastic-backed absorbent pads under connections. If a closed system is not available, wrap sterile gauze around the tubing connection to reduce the potential for spraying or leaking of drug into the environment when attaching or removing the tubing or syringe.

Table 6. Oral Hazardous Drug Formulation Categories and Avenues of Exposure During Preparation and Administration

Preparation	Comments	Safety Measure	Avenues of HD Exposure	Considerations
Liquids	Preferred formulation for gastrostomy tube administration because the drug is readily absorbed and less likely to cause tube clogging	Oral HD-filled syringes must be labeled as NG-HD. Do not administer suspension macrogranules or mineral oil in nasogastric tubes.	**Preparation:** When the drug is dispensed in a granule- or powder-filled package, it requires reconstitution or dilution. **Administration:** Leakage during transfer of liquids from their bottles to administration syringe system.	High concentration of sorbitol in drug formulation; check with pharmacist or package insert. When reconstitution or dissolution occurs, consult with pharmacy to determine if there is a specific time frame that the preparation must be administered due to stability issues. Manufacture challenges to create and/or adapt closed transfer systems. Adaptation of pediatric bottle-syringe transfer systems. Use of Luer-lock syringe devices will necessitate the adaptation of tube designs and/or conversion systems to accommodate Luer-locking systems.
Suspension	Lower sorbitol concentration compared to liquids	High osmolality, requiring diluting with water to decrease the tonicity	**Preparation:** Transfer leakage from bottle to administration syringes. **Administration:** Leakage at the tube-syringe site.	Not many HDs come in suspension formulation (e.g., megestrol, mycophenolate mofetil, valganciclovir). Manufacture challenges to create and/or adapt closed transfer systems. Adaptation of pediatric bottle-syringe transfer systems. Use of Luer-lock syringe devices will necessitate the adaptation of tube designs and/or conversion systems to accommodate Luer-locking systems.
Immediate release (i.e., compressed tablets, sugar- or film-coated)	Crushing minimizes pharmacokinetic changes and is considered more beneficial than some of the liquid formulations.	Minimal pharmacokinetic changes	**Preparation:** Fine powder manipulation with mortar and pestle results in equipment and surface contamination and aerosolization. Leakage is likely when transferring solutions into administration syringe. Some techniques exist for dissolving the tablet within the syringe. **Administration:** Exposure occurs because of "powder" particulate aerosolization and surface contamination. Leakage at the abdominal tube insertion site related to poor wound healing, ascites, etc., resulting in linen/dressing contamination.	When reconstitution or dissolution occurs, consult with pharmacy to determine if there is a specific time frame that the preparation must be administered due to stability issues (e.g., cyclophosphamide, gefitinib). Manufacture challenges to create and/or adapt closed transfer systems. Adaptation of pediatric bottle-syringe transfer systems. Use of Luer-lock syringe devices will necessitate the adaptation of tube designs and/or conversion systems to accommodate Luer-locking systems.

(Continued on next page)

Table 6. Oral Hazardous Drug Formulation Categories and Avenues of Exposure During Preparation and Administration *(Continued)*

Preparation	Comments	Safety Measure	Avenues of HD Exposure	Considerations
Enteric-coated tablet	DO NOT CRUSH.	Medication will be released in the small intestine instead of the stomach. This will result in increased toxicity profile. Crushing will also cause tube clogging.	N/A	N/A
Extended-release powder-filled capsule	DO NOT CRUSH. Capsule may be opened to administer powder through a feeding tube.	Crushing destroys the delivery mechanism and can result in toxic effects.	**Preparation with powder:** Opening the capsule may cause powder aerosolization and surface contamination.	N/A: currently no HD extended-release formulation
Powder-filled capsule	DO NOT CRUSH.		**Preparation:** Open the capsule in a BSC. If the BSC is unavailable, then PPE with an N57 mask should be used. Once the powder is reconstituted, leakage is likely when transferring solutions into administration syringe. **Administration:** Leakage at the tube-syringe site. Leakage at the abdominal tube insertion site related to poor wound healing, ascites, etc., resulting in linen/dressing contamination.	N/A
Gel-filled capsule	DO NOT CRUSH.	Soft gelatin capsule generally contains a pharmaceutical dissolved or dispersed in a carrier that is compatible with the capsule wall. In addition to liquids, the fill material may take the form of a semisolid, solid, or gel.	**Preparation:** To be performed by pharmacy. **Administration:** Leakage at the tube-syringe site. Leakage at the abdominal tube insertion site related to poor wound healing, ascites, etc., resulting in linen/dressing contamination.	N/A
Buccal or sublingual	DO NOT CRUSH.	Not designed for gastrointestinal absorption, thereby reducing efficacy	N/A	N/A

BSC—biologic safety cabinet; HD—hazardous drug; N/A—not applicable; NG—nasogastric; PPE—personal protective equipment

Note. Based on information from Mitchell, 2010; Occupational Safety and Health Administration, 1995; Williams, 2008.

Figure 7. Washburn Setup

Setup for Tube Administration

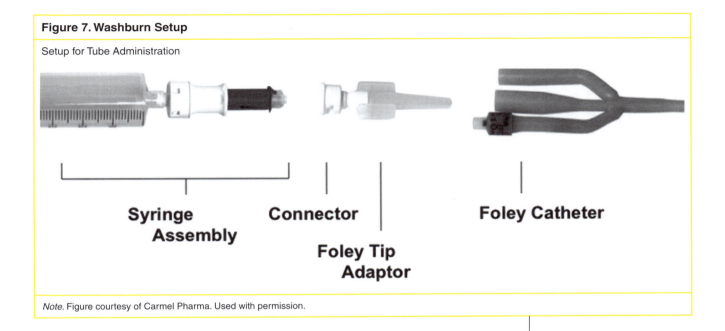

Syringe Assembly | Connector | Foley Tip Adaptor | Foley Catheter

Note. Figure courtesy of Carmel Pharma. Used with permission.

Intravesicular Administration

Intravesicular HD administration is performed using a Foley catheter placed in the bladder for direct instillation. This type of treatment is used for patients with transitional cell cancer or urothelial bladder cancer (Raghavan, 2009). The HD is usually delivered using a catheter-tip syringe placed into an empty bladder. A suprapubic catheter inserted through the pubic wall into the bladder also may be used to deliver HDs into the bladder. The type of catheter used will determine the type of connection needed for safe administration.

Begin by emptying the bladder and drainage bag of all urine. Use the Washburn (2007) setup if possible. Place a plastic-backed absorbent pad under connections. While wearing PPE, administer the HD into the bladder using the Foley catheter followed by a normal saline flush. Clamp the Foley catheter. If ordered, instruct the patient to rotate from side to side to increase distribution of the drug solution to the entire bladder cavity. After the ordered dwell time, unclamp the Foley catheter and let the HD-contaminated fluid drain into the closed gravity-dependent Foley bag system. Handle the urinary drainage as contaminated body fluid, wearing double chemotherapy gloves, a chemotherapy gown, and a face shield if indicated. Prudent practice dictates that the Foley catheter itself should be discarded similarly.

Intraperitoneal Delivery

Intraperitoneal (IP) delivery is a type of intracavitary administration of HD into the peritoneum. Indications for IP administration include colon cancer, cytoreduced ovarian cancer, appendiceal cancer, sarcomas, peritoneal carcinomatosis or sarcomatosis, and malignant ascites (Cannistra, Gershenson, & Recht, 2008; Hydrik, 2009; Libutti, Saltz, & Tepper, 2008; NCI, 2006).

The peritoneum is a physiologic barrier to drugs administered parenterally or orally. Exposure of peritoneal surfaces to pharmacologically active drugs can be increased considerably by direct administration via the IP route (Sugarbaker, 1998). This type of HD delivery results in high drug concentrations and longer drug half-life in the peritoneal cavity, thus increasing local effects of the drugs (Pingpank, 2008; Sugarbaker, Klecker, Gianola, & Speyer, 1986).

IP HDs are delivered through an IP implanted port where the catheter tip is located directly in the peritoneal cavity. The port device is placed subcutaneously over the lower ribs. The attached catheter is either fenestrated (multiple holes along the distal half of the catheter in addition to the distal opening) or standard (with only the distal end open). This device may be placed during surgery or using fluoroscopy in interventional radiology (Rundback et al., 1994). Use IV tubing with a Luer-lock or a closed-system connection. Anchor the needle securely to the port septum. Check the patency of the port system by flushing with sterile normal saline. If there is no resistance, proceed with administration.

A fenestrated Tenckhoff peritoneal dialysis catheter also may be used for peritoneal HD delivery. It is an external catheter that is inserted through the abdominal wall into the peritoneal cavity. A Dacron cuff reduces peritoneal leaking and bacterial tracking (Rundback et al., 1994). When using an external catheter for IP drug delivery, use an adapter that will accommodate a locking connection.

While wearing PPE, place a plastic-backed absorbent pad under connections. Infuse the drug solution. Once the infusion is complete, follow the physician's order regarding patient positioning and dwell time. If the infused solution is to be drained, leave the administration set connected. After drug delivery and prescribed dwell time (if applicable), withdraw or drain the residual solution. Handle the residual solution as contaminated body fluid.

Intrapleural Administration

HD administered through the chest wall into the pleural space is indicated for malignant pleural effusions (MPEs) caused by mesotheliomas, carcinoma of the lung, breast cancer, lymphomas, ovarian cancer, and gastrointestinal tract cancers. MPE treatments include repeated thoracentesis, chemical sclerosing, talc pleurodesis, and HD administration. Long-term intrapleural catheter placement (i.e., chest tube, pigtail catheter, fenestrated portacath [Driesen et al., 1994; Shoji, Tanaka, Yanagihara, Inui, & Wada, 2002], Tenckhoff catheters [Walker & Bryden, 2010]), and a temporary thoracentesis needle can be used for fluid removal and HD administration. These placement procedures may be performed at the bedside, intraoperatively, or in interventional radiology.

While wearing PPE, place a plastic-backed absorbent pad under connections. Infuse the drug solution. Once the infusion is complete, follow the physician's order regarding patient positioning and dwell time. If the infused solution is to be drained, leave the administration set connected. After drug delivery and prescribed dwell time (if applicable), withdraw or drain the residual solution. Handle the residual solution as contaminated body fluid.

When using a chest tube (with and without collection device), portacath, or Tenckhoff catheter, use IV tubing with closed-system or locking connections. After drug delivery and prescribed dwell time, attach the drainage apparatus to the connection and lower it to collect the residual solution. If the catheter tubing has a female opening, consider adaptation of the Washburn setup as shown in Figure 7.

Handle the residual solution as contaminated body fluid, wearing a gown, gloves, and face shield. Dispose of all materials used in the administration as hazardous waste. Remove PPE, seal in plastic bag, and dispose of in appropriate container. Don gloves and decontaminate equipment used during administration. Wash hands thoroughly.

Aerosolized or Inhaled Administration

Aerosol delivery is the administration of HDs via particles that are inhaled and absorbed through the lungs. Aerosol drug administration may be referred to as *inhalation* or *nebulized therapy*. Aerosols include metered dose inhaler systems, dry powder inhalers, and nebulizers for delivery of high concentrations of HDs locally while minimizing systemic toxicity. The target areas for delivery are the pulmonary system (Kaparissides, Alexandridou, Kotti, & Chaitidou, 2006) and the central nervous system (CNS). When administering aerosolized HDs, the HCW must wear a NIOSH-approved respirator (ASHP, 2006; OSHA, 1995; Tatsumura, Koyama, Tsujimoto, Kitagawa, & Kagamimori, 1993; Welch & Silveira, 1997; Wittgen et al., 2007). Coordinate the procedure with the safety officer or respiratory therapist (Sutton, 2004). Inhalation of HDs should take place in a negative pressure room using a closed inhalation system that isolates the patient in a vinyl enclosure similar to an oxygen tent. Air is drawn upward from the area inside the canopy and flows through a HEPA filter. Don PPE including respirator, gown, gloves, cap, and shoe covers when aerosolized HDs are present because aerosols may be deposited on skin and surfaces.

Implanted Time-Release Delivery

The chance of occupational exposure to nanoparticles has not been addressed, but is possible due to the particle size (Stern & McNeil, 2008). A thin film polymer sandwich of nanodiamonds clustered with HDs, RNA, or other targeting material is placed in a tumor bed following tumor removal or debulking. This delivery system allows drug release to a specific location (Ho, 2008; Kunwar et al., 2007; Mardor et al., 2005). An example of this is the use of polymer wafers in the treatment of brain tumors (polifeprosan 20 with carmustine implant, Gliadel®, Eisai Inc.). These HD-impregnated wafers are placed intraoperatively following tumor debulking. The surgical team wears surgical chemotherapy gloves when handling the wafer during implantation and disposes of the wafer packaging in an HD waste container. Refer to the package insert to determine duration of drug release and length of time to use precautions after placement.

Intraventricular, Intrathecal, Intraspinal, and Intracerebral Administration

The blood-brain barrier (BBB) significantly limits drug penetration into the CNS when drugs are administered by the parenteral or oral route (Batchelor & Supko, 2009; Brown & Meyers, 2008; Larson, Rubenstein, & McDermott, 2008; Margolin & Poplack, 2008; Mehta, Buckner, Sawaya, & Cannon, 2008; Patel, 2007; Sampson et al., 2006). A number of delivery methods are designed to allow HDs to cross the BBB. These systems include intraventricular, intrathecal, intra-arterial, intracerebral, convection-enhanced delivery procedure and device, and interstitial.

The intraventricular and intrathecal routes are methods used to deliver HDs into the cerebrospinal fluid (CSF). Indications for administration of HD via these routes include CNS carcinomatosis, leptomeningeal metastasis, and CNS leukemic infiltrates (Aiello-Laws & Rutledge, 2008; Baehring, 2008; Batchelor & Supko, 2009; DeAngelis & Yahalom, 2008; Patel, 2007; Sampson et al., 2006).

Intrathecal HD administration is delivered through a lumbar puncture by a credentialed physician or advanced practitioner. To prevent increased CSF pressure, a small volume of CSF equal to the volume of drug is removed. The

HD-filled syringe is attached to a spinal needle, and the HD is slowly injected. The provider dons PPE and places a plastic-backed absorbent pad under the site where the needle enters the spine and the syringe connection. The lumbar puncture is an invasive and sterile procedure. Sterile chemotherapy gloves should be worn. The lumbar needle and infusion system should be discarded in an HD waste container.

If an epidural catheter is used for the intrathecal delivery system, the catheter can be accessed for intermittent bolus administration or be attached to an infusion pump. Access and administration using these delivery systems may be performed by credentialed advanced practitioners or RNs who have demonstrated clinical competence for this procedure. Recommended precautions are the same as for IV HD administration.

An implanted reservoir (Ommaya reservoir) may be placed surgically or in interventional radiology. It is a silicone reservoir placed subcutaneously in the scalp that can be used to deliver HDs into the ventricles. HD administration using an implanted reservoir is performed by a physician, an advanced practitioner, or an RN with demonstrated clinical competence, depending on the nurse practice act or local policy. When accessing the implanted reservoir, use a closed system or Luer-lock connection to a Huber needle-tubing system. Wear double chemotherapy gloves, a chemotherapy gown, and a face shield if indicated. Handle CSF fluid as contaminated, and dispose of all materials used in the administration as hazardous waste.

An interstitial CNS drug delivery system circumvents the BBB, resulting in higher HD concentrations with minimal systemic exposure and toxicity. Three categories of interstitial CNS delivery systems exist based on the infusion mechanism of the pumps. The catheters can be placed in the epidural space or intracranially. These pumps may be implanted for external attachment and are as follows.

- The Infusaid™ Pump (Infusaid Corp.) uses compressed pressure generated from Freon® (DuPont) gas vapor to deliver HDs at a constant rate.
- The MiniMed™ Programmable Implantable Infusion System (MiniMed Technologies) uses a solenoid pumping mechanism.
- The SynchroMed® (Medtronic) drug delivery system uses a peristaltic mechanism.

Please note that these pumps may also be used for other HD delivery applications (i.e., intra-arterial). Accessing and refilling these delivery systems may be performed only by credentialed physicians, advanced practitioners, or RNs who have demonstrated clinical competence for this procedure. PPE is required as for IV administration.

Intraocular Administration

HDs may be administered into the eye, by either subconjunctival or intravitreal administration (de Smet, Vancs, Kohler, Solomon, & Chan, 1999; Gangaputra, Nussenblatt, & Levy-Clarke, 2008). This type of procedure is performed by a credentialed practitioner or ophthalmologist for refractory or recurrent intraocular parenchymal or leptomeningeal lymphoma (de Smet et al., 1999), retinoblastoma (Hayden et al., 2004; Mulvihill et al., 2003), and ocular Behçet disease (Atmaca-Sonmez, Atmaca, & Aydintug, 2007).

The HD is prepared in a syringe for injection. The provider should wear double chemotherapy gloves, a chemotherapy gown, and a face shield if indicated. Drape the patient to contain leakage. Handle any drainage as contaminated body fluid and dispose of all materials used in the administration as HD waste.

Intra-Arterial Delivery

HDs may be administered into an artery that is the primary blood supply to a tumor. Angiography is performed to visualize the vessels that supply the tumor. A catheter is placed and advanced into the identified artery. The HD is administered, exposing the tumor to high drug concentrations with significant reduction in systemic toxicities. One of the goals of this procedure may also be to occlude the arteries feeding the tumor. This procedure is used for primary hepatocellular carcinoma, head and neck cancers, and solitary hepatic metastases from other primary tumors (Roth et al., 2000).

Percutaneous Administration

Femoral, brachial, or carotid vessels are the most common arteries accessed. The hepatic arteries are the most common vessels entered. Percutaneous administration may represent a significant opportunity for exposure because of bleeding at the puncture site and because the drug delivery equipment used may not be designed to protect HCWs. Use a CSTD or locking connections whenever possible. Wear double sterile chemotherapy gloves, a sterile impermeable gown, and a face shield if indicated. Sterile gloves must be changed every 30 minutes for lengthy procedures (Singleton & Connor, 1999; Wallemacq et al., 2006). Place plastic-backed absorbent pads under the patient. Wrap sterile gauze around the connection to reduce the potential for spraying or leaking of the drug into the environment when attaching or removing the tubing or syringe. Dispose of all materials used in the administration as HD waste. Note: If HDs are transferred from vials or other systems in the procedural suite, the transfer must be performed using closed systems to prevent aerosolized exposure of staff. If closed systems are unavailable, then all staff must wear an approved respirator (ASHP, 2006; Matthews, Snell, & Coats, 2006; Muehlbauer et al., 2006; NIOSH, 2004; OSHA, 1995).

Continuous Infusion Via Intra-Arterial Placed Pump

HDs may be delivered intra-arterially through an implanted pump (e.g., Infusaid, SynchroMed) by credentialed nurses with a clinical competence for this procedure, advanced practitioners, or physicians. When accessing or using the intra-arterial infusion pump, use a closed or Luer-locking connection and a Huber needle-tubing system. Don double chemotherapy gloves, a gown, and a face shield if indicated. Place plastic-backed absorbent pads under the connection. Wrap sterile gauze around the connection to reduce the potential for spraying or leaking of the drug into the environment when attaching or removing the tubing or syringe. Once the procedure is completed, dispose of the administration equipment as HD waste.

Nontraditional Settings for Hazardous Drug Delivery

HD handling can occur in many healthcare settings. The opportunities for HCW exposure to HDs in alternative settings are related to the type of procedures performed. Some procedures may involve administration of HDs. Some procedures may be performed for patients who have recently received HDs, and their body fluids are a source of exposure. Precautions are necessary to avoid exposure while handling patients' contaminated excreta, including blood, urine, feces, tissue specimens, effusions, and all bodily fluids. It is essential that nurses communicate with personnel in these settings where patients are cared for, so that they will be aware of the potential for HD exposure. The staff in these settings may not be trained in the use of HD safe handling precautions. Non-nursing staff may be involved with the handling and/or processing of body fluids and tissue and need to be informed that the materials or substances require handling precautions.

Some examples of nontraditional settings for HD administration include

- Radiology department
- Pulmonary laboratory (e.g., during bronchoscopy)
- Nuclear medicine departments
- Computed tomography/magnetic resonance imaging locations (i.e., biopsies)
- Gastrointestinal laboratory (e.g., during endoscopy or sigmoid-colonoscopy)
- Cardiac catheterization laboratory/suites
- Radiation therapy department
- Ultrasound/sonography department (e.g., effusion removal [centesis], fluid pocket aspirations, biopsies)
- Skilled nursing facilities and long-term care facilities
- Rehabilitation facilities
- Homecare settings
- Hemodialysis department
- Pheresis department
- Operating room (OR)
- Veterinary clinics and hospitals
- Pharmacy mini-clinics
- Clinical laboratories
- Camps and schools.

Dialysis and Pheresis

When patients receiving HDs undergo hemodialysis, it is strongly recommended that the HD administration be coordinated with the nephrologist and hemodialysis RN. Any staff involved in patient care must wear chemotherapy-designated PPE when disposing of the dialysate solution and tubing. The hemodialysis equipment must be decontaminated prior to its next use or removal from the patient care setting.

Apheresis is a procedure that involves removing whole blood and separating it into individual components so that a particular component can be removed. The remaining blood components then are reinfused into the bloodstream of the patient or donor. Apheresis is used for the collection of donor blood components as well as for the treatment of certain medical conditions. Screen the patient's or donor's medication list for use of HDs within the past 48 hours. Use HD safe handling precautions during the procedure. Consider all disposable equipment contaminated, and discard it in an HD waste container. Decontaminate all nondisposable equipment after use.

Operative and Interventional Settings

When HDs are administered intraoperatively, it is necessary for the rooms to be prepared prior to the patient's arrival. Place absorbent pads on the OR table to absorb HD-contaminated fluids that may leak during the procedure. Place absorbent pads on the floor between the setup table and the OR table. This is a high-traffic area for the medical, nursing, and technician team preparing medications, guidewires, and other instrumentation. Fluids that leak on the floor could potentially be tracked elsewhere on the shoe covers of the OR team (Connor & Eisenberg, 2010). Dispose of all fluid collection devices (i.e., nasogastric, Foley, suction drains) and surgical sponges as HD waste. Coordinate HD drug preparation with the pharmacy. Using a CSTD will minimize HD leakage and aerosolization (Foltz, Wavrin, & Sticca, 2004; Muehlbauer et al., 2006).

Decontaminate reusable equipment (Muehlbauer et al., 2006). Handle tissue specimens as contaminated items. Make sure that recovery staff wears PPE when coming in contact with the patient and any excreta for at least 48 hours. If the patient is discharged home, inform the family and caretakers about the appropriate precautions for handling excreta. Examples of some types of intraoperative procedures include

- Isolated limb perfusion for extremity sarcomas or melanomas (Brennan, Singer, Maki, & O'Sullivan, 2008; Matthews et al., 2006)
- Isolated hepatic perfusion (Bartlett, Bisceglie, & Dawson, 2008; Brown & Meyers, 2008; Muehlbauer et al., 2006; Sugarbaker, 1998)
- Intraoperative IP HD administration
  - Intraoperative closed technique: Following cytoreduction, inflow and outflow catheters are placed. Following temporary closure of the abdomen, the chemotherapy solution is infused. The abdominal wall is manually agitated during the perfusion period to promote uniform infusate distribution. At the completion of the perfusion, the abdomen is reopened, and the solution is evacuated.
  - Open abdomen technique (coliseum technique): Inflow and outflow catheters are placed as described. A silastic sheet is sutured over a retractor and to the patient's skin, over the abdominal opening. This creates a container for the instillation of the chemotherapy infusate.
  - Hyperthermic IP chemotherapy: Following cytoreductive surgery, a Tenckhoff catheter and closed suction drains are placed through the abdominal wall and made watertight with purse-string sutures at the skin. Temperature probes are secured into the skin. The skin edges are then sutured to the self-retaining retractor, and a plastic sheet is incorporated into these sutures to create an open space beneath using the coliseum technique. During a 1-½ hour perfusion, all the peritoneal anatomic structures are uniformly exposed to heat and chemotherapy. The surgeon vigorously manipulates all viscera to minimize peritoneal adherence. A heat exchanger keeps the circulating fluid at 44°–46°C. A smoke evacuator is used to pull air from beneath the plastic cover through activated charcoal, reducing aerosols in the OR suite. Following completion of the intraoperative perfusion, the abdomen is suctioned and surgically closed (Foltz et al., 2004; Sugarbaker, 1998; Sugarbaker et al., 1986; Yan, Stuart, Yoo, & Sugarbaker, 2006).

Post-Administration Issues

Body Fluids

Variable amounts of HDs and their metabolites are excreted in the urine, stool, sweat, and other body excreta of patients receiving HDs. As an example, up to 30% of an IV dose of cyclophosphamide is excreted unchanged in the urine within two days of administration (ASHP, 2009; Thomson Reuters Micromedex® 2.0, 2009). Not all references agree on elimination data, and variables such as infusion rate and renal function can influence how long active drug or metabolites are present in stool and urine. Although information is not available for all drugs, two days (48 hours) has been recommended as a time frame for use of HD precautions when handling body fluids because the majority of drugs are excreted within this time (ASHP, 1990; OSHA, 1995). Drugs falling outside of that window are presented in Table 7. Some practice settings may prefer to adapt drug-specific time frames for instituting protective precautions, whereas others may opt to simplify by using one time frame for all HDs. Organizations using computerized physician order entry

Table 7. Hazardous Drugs Requiring Personal Protection for Longer Than Two Days

Hazardous Drug	Detected in Urine	Detected in Stool or Bile
Carmustine	At least 4 days	–
Cisplatin	At least 5 days	–
Docetaxel	6% excretion	Up to 7 days
Doxorubicin	5% excretion for up to 5 days	Up to 7 days
Etoposide	At least 5 days	–
Gemcitabine	At least 7 days	–
Imatinib mesylate	13% excretion for up to 7 days	Up to 7 days
Methotrexate (oral)	Up to 5 days	Up to 5 days
Mitoxantrone	Up to 5 days	Up to 5 days
Temsirolimus	4.6% excretion for up to 14 days	78% excretion for up to 14 days
Teniposide	Up to 5 days	–
Vincristine	Minimal excretion	Up to 3 days
Vinorelbine	Minimal excretion	At least 3 days

Note. Based on information from American Society of Health-System Pharmacists, 2009; Thomson Reuters Micromedex® 2.0, 2009.

Figure 8. Some Hazardous Drugs Known to Be Secreted in Breast Milk

- Arsenic trioxide
- Cisplatin
- Cyclophosphamide
- Cyclosporine
- Doxorubicin
- Etoposide
- Exemestane
- Goserelin
- Imatinib
- Interferon alfa-2b
- Lomustine
- Megestrol acetate
- Mercaptopurine
- Methotrexate
- Mitomycin
- Mitoxantrone
- Streptozocin
- Tacrolimus
- Tretinoin
- Vincristine
- Zidovudine

Note. Based on information from Turkoski et al., 2009.

may add information about the duration of precautions to orders for specific HDs.

Other exceptions to the duration of the precautions may occur. One of these is the presence of effusions. HDs have been measured in peritoneal and pleural effusions (Gotlieb et al., 2007; Pestieau, Schnake, Stuart, & Sugarbaker, 2001; Shoji et al., 2002; Sugarbaker & Stephens, n.d.; Van der Speeten, Stuart, Mahteme, & Sugarbaker, 2009; Yulan et al., 2003). This has implications for invasive procedures, such as paracentesis, thoracentesis, or pericardiocentesis. In addition, nanoformulations of drugs also extend or delay HD release or activation (Muehlbauer et al., 2006; Muthu & Singh, 2009). HD residue may be present longer, necessitating use of precautions for extended periods of time.

Some HDs are secreted in breast milk. Although information about drug secretion in breast milk is often unknown, it is available for some HDs (see Figure 8). Nursing infants may receive up to 10% of the maternal dose of imatinib (Gleevec® [Novartis Pharmaceuticals Corp., 2009]). It is also possible for some drugs to be present in higher concentrations in breast milk than in serum. For example, although information about human lactation is not known, the concentration of sunitinib (Sutent® [Pfizer Inc., 2010]) in rat breast milk is 12 times higher than in serum. Nurses should consider this possibility when making decisions about handling HDs while breast-feeding.

HDs may be present in emesis following oral administration. Methotrexate also has been measured in the emesis of patients who received it intravenously (Mader et al., 1996). HDs have been measured in the sweat of patients receiving high doses of methotrexate (Mader et al., 1996) and other HDs administered in myeloablative doses. Cyclophosphamide has been found in the seminal fluid of rats (Hales, Smith, & Robaire, 1986).

HCWs should use recommended PPE for two days after completion of therapy when handling the body fluids or linens of patients who have received HDs. The same PPE used for administering HDs should be worn whenever handling body fluids, particularly urine, of a patient who has received the drugs (Polovich et al., 2009). A face shield must be worn whenever splashing is possible.

Published surveys have demonstrated poor compliance of HCWs for wearing PPE while handling excreta of patients being treated with HDs (Martin & Larson, 2003; Nieweg et al., 1994). When nurses do not follow standard precautions, they place themselves at risk for exposure (Connor & McDiarmid, 2006).

Some hospitals and clinics post a sign in the patient's bathroom alerting nurses and ancillary staff to use PPE when emptying excreta. This may be particularly useful for staff who are not aware that the patient has received chemotherapy.

No published research has established the effectiveness of double flushing for reducing HD contamination. Some hospital toilets use powerful, high-pressure flushing mechanisms, and many do not have a lid, which can potentially result in aerosolization during flushing. Some facilities require the toilet to be covered with a plastic-backed absorbent pad while flushing. The HCW should wear PPE while handling the pad and dispose of it properly.

Double flushing at home may be useful in situations where there is insufficient volume or pressure to clear the toilet after use (Polovich et al., 2009). Nurses should discuss the topic with patients prior to discharge and ultimately allow them to determine whether the additional flush is warranted. When family members handle patients' contaminated excreta, they should wear gloves.

In addition to donning PPE, nurses and supportive personnel should consider other ways to reduce exposure to HDs found in body fluids. Such measures may include

- Using patients' weights rather than intake and output to monitor fluid status
- Weighing urinary output collected in drainage bags rather than measuring volume to reduce the risk of splashing when transferring urine into a second container before disposal
- Encouraging men to sit on toilet seats rather than standing to reduce the risk of droplet contamination
- Encouraging use of toilets rather than urinals and bedpans when feasible to decrease the possibility of spillage
- When applicable, collecting drainage of pleural, peritoneal, and other body fluids in a closed system that can be disposed of intact
- If possible, using disposable ostomy pouches rather than rinsing and reusing them
- Protecting the skin of incontinent patients from their own excreta. The metabolites of drugs found in the urine or stool may be damaging to the skin. Cleanse the skin with soap and water and apply a moisture barrier to the perineal and perirectal areas following each urination or stool. Apply a clean disposable diaper.
- Using a Vacutainer® (Becton, Dickinson and Co.) system when collecting blood samples to reduce the chance of blood exposure when transferring blood from a syringe to a specimen tube.

Linen Handling

Linens contaminated with HDs pose a health risk for HCWs, family members, and other caregivers who come in contact with them. While the HD exposure may be less when handling contaminated linens than when handling a drug during the preparation and administration phases, some drugs are excreted unchanged in the urine and the safe level of HD exposure is unknown. When considering linen handling, two main considerations exist. First, there is a need to prevent linen contamination. Second, linens contaminated with HDs should be handled safely to reduce occupational exposure and workplace contamination.

Figure 9 identifies ways to reduce the contamination of linens with HDs. These methods focus on using disposable items and fabrics that are less permeable to fluids than traditional cloth linens. Particular attention should be paid to these practices when patients are incontinent. Disposable items that are contaminated with even trace amounts of HDs should be discarded as HD waste (OSHA, 2002).

In the event that linens do become contaminated with HDs as a result of an HD spill or contact with body fluids that may contain residual HDs because of incontinence, vomiting, or diaphoresis, the linens require spe-

---

Figure 9. Ways to Reduce Linen Contamination With Hazardous Drugs

- For incontinent patients, both children and adults, disposable, plastic-backed, leak-resistant diapers are preferred to cloth diapers that are intended for washing and reuse.
- Use plastic- or vinyl-covered pillows rather than cloth-covered pillows to make cleaning easier in the case of hazardous drug contamination.
- Discourage the use of bedpans and bedside urinals, which are prone to spilling. Instead, encourage ambulatory patients to use the bathroom facilities.
- Use plastic- or vinyl-treated chairs that can be easily decontaminated rather than upholstered chairs that cannot be readily cleaned.

cial handling. OSHA (1995) specifies that linens contaminated with HDs should be double bagged, first in a specially marked bag and then in labeled impervious bags. In the laundry facility, the outer impervious bag should be removed and discarded after the inner bag containing the contaminated linens is placed directly into the washing machine. The laundry bag and contents should be prewashed alone before a second washing with other laundry (OSHA, 1995). The current handling recommendations from NIOSH specify that workers who handle linens of patients who have received HDs in the past 48 hours, and in some instances for up to seven days, should wear two pairs of disposable gloves and a disposable gown (NIOSH, 2004).

Some hospitals and laundry services do not require the HD-contaminated laundry to be double bagged because they treat all linens as potentially hazardous or biohazardous waste. To that end, they double wash and bleach all linens, and laundry personnel don full PPE for handling all linens. OSHA (2002) requires employers to ensure that employees wear appropriate PPE, such as gloves, gowns, face shields, and masks, when handling linens contaminated with blood-borne pathogens. OSHA does not set specific standards for handling linens contaminated with HDs, instead referring to the standard on blood-borne pathogens (OSHA, 1992/2008). In organizations where all laundry is handled as contaminated, the laundry must be bagged in an impervious bag to prevent environmental contamination resulting from soak-through and leakage. Nurses working in settings where all linen waste is not double bagged should investigate to ensure that appropriate care is being taken in the laundry department to protect the employees and the environment.

The current standard for handling HD-contaminated linens is to adhere to recommendations in the blood-borne pathogens standard as described previously. The Association for Linen Management (formerly the National Association of Institutional Linen Management), however, proposes strict double bagging of all hospital laundry of patients who have received HDs in the past 48 hours (up to seven days in specific instances). The association proposes a three-step process that includes recognizing potentially contaminated linen, education and training, and work practice recommendations. The proposal specifies that HD-contaminated linens should not be mixed with biohazardous (red-bagged) linens and that a separate color code should be used to designate the linens as hazardous (Association for Linen Management, 2009).

For most patients receiving HDs, home linens can be handled the same as other household laundry. Special handling should be implemented if an HD spill occurs in the home or if laundry becomes contaminated with the excreta of the person receiving HDs. In the home, patients should handle their own contaminated linens when feasible. Family members or caregivers should don chemotherapy gowns and double gloves if they are handling contaminated linens. Contaminated linens in the home should be double washed with hot water and detergent separately from other household laundry. Bleach should be used when feasible, considering the fabric, for its role in deactivating HDs. Whenever possible, the contaminated items should be placed directly into the washing machine to avoid contamination of any intermediary storage container. If the contaminated laundry cannot be washed immediately, placing the items in a plastic bag prevents contamination of a laundry basket or storage container. The plastic bag should be disposed of immediately in the household trash after the linens are placed in the washing machine to prevent spreading contamination. A common-sense approach to handling HD-contaminated linen will prevent further environmental contamination in both the homecare and healthcare settings.

Disposal of Hazardous Drugs

Hazardous waste must be handled separately from other medical waste to ensure that those individuals handling the waste are protected from potential exposure and to safeguard the environment. The Medical Waste Tracking Act of 1988 defined medical waste as "any solid waste that is generated in the diagnosis, treatment, or immunization of human beings or animals, in research pertaining thereto, or in the production or testing of biologicals" (U.S. Environmental Protection Agency [EPA], 2010a). Medical waste includes infectious ("red-bag") and noninfectious waste. It refers to biologic substances or wastes that come in contact with biologic substances.

Hazardous waste is defined by the EPA in the Resource Conservation and Recovery Act (RCRA) as waste that may "(i) Cause, or significantly contribute to, an increase in mortality or an increase in serious irreversible or incapacitating reversible illness; or (ii) pose a substantial present or potential hazard to human health or the environment when it is improperly treated, stored, transported, disposed of, or otherwise managed" (U.S. EPA, 2009).

It is important to note that the term *hazardous drug* refers to risks to employees and is regulated by OSHA, and *hazardous waste* refers to risks to the environment and is regulated by the EPA. While some overlap exists, not all HDs are currently regulated as hazardous waste although they probably should be. Likewise, a number of common drugs, such as warfarin, are hazardous to the environment but are not a risk to HCWs. These are regulated as hazardous waste but do not require PPE for administration. Figure 10 provides an example of the two sets of definitions.

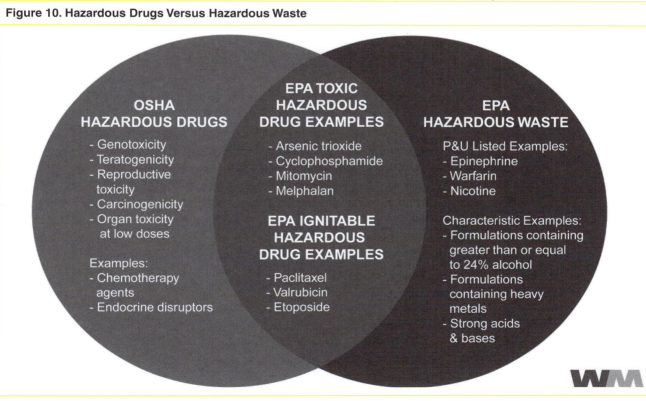

Figure 10. Hazardous Drugs Versus Hazardous Waste

EPA—U.S. Environmental Protection Agency; OSHA—Occupational Safety and Health Administration

Note. Copyright 2010 by WM Healthcare Solutions, Inc. Used with permission.

Hazardous wastes are defined in several ways by the EPA and are divided into *listed* wastes and *characteristic* waste. Listed wastes are given P codes (acutely hazardous) and U codes (toxic), among others. The only P-listed chemotherapy agent is arsenic trioxide. Several chemotherapy drugs are U-listed (chlorambucil, cyclophosphamide, daunorubicin, diethylstilbestrol, melphalan, mitomycin C, streptozocin), meaning that they possess one or more of the following characteristics: toxicity, ignitability, corrosivity, or reactivity. Managing hazardous wastes is a relatively complex process and requires "cradle to grave" tracking and incineration at a hazardous waste facility. Hospital safety officers or environmental services managers need to be heavily involved in implementing a pharmaceutical waste program. Many other HDs have characteristics similar to the original listed drugs. Although the EPA has not updated the list in more than 30 years, best management practices are to manage these drugs as hazardous waste based on their toxicity.

HD waste containers must be available in all areas where HDs are prepared and administered (OSHA, 1995). The waste containers should be puncture-proof, have a lid that seals securely, and be labeled with an appropriate warning. The warning label identifies the contents as "Hazardous Waste" so that the individuals transporting the waste are alerted to the need for special handling. The container should be distinctly different from other types of waste containers (such as those used for infectious waste) and should be used only for HD waste (ASHP, 1990, 2006; NIOSH, 2004; OSHA, 1995). Plastic bags may be used to contain hazardous waste, such as the sealable bag that is used for drug transport, but these should then be placed inside a rigid waste container. Keep the lid closed on hazardous waste containers except for when placing waste into the containers. These practices reduce the risk of drug vapors being released into the environment, as has been described by Connor et al. (2000). This practice also meets hazardous waste regulations for containment. Several container manufacturers provide black hazardous waste containers designed for use in healthcare settings to differentiate them from other types of wastes.

When HCWs are dealing with chemotherapy, any item that has come into contact with an HD during its preparation or administration is considered to be "trace contaminated." Although it is not regulated in all states, the best management practice is to segregate these items into a separate waste stream, typically using a yellow container, and have them incinerated as regulated medical waste. This ensures they are not autoclaved with red-bag waste and also enables needles and other sharps to be properly disposed. Combining needles and other sharps with hazardous waste creates a dual biohazardous/hazardous waste stream, which is very expensive to dispose of.

Disposal requirements are less stringent when a container is considered "empty" under RCRA. Therefore, HCWs must be able to determine whether a container that held a listed waste is "RCRA-empty." For a P-listed drug, such as arsenic trioxide, the container is never empty because of an EPA requirement that all containers that have held a P-listed waste must be triple rinsed to be considered empty (U.S. EPA, 2010b). Because that is not practical in health care, all ampoules or IVs that contained arsenic trioxide must be disposed as hazardous waste. The only exception is an exclusion EPA granted in April 2008 for a used syringe (U.S. EPA, 2008). For HDs that are U-listed or exhibit one of the criteria of a hazardous waste, such as ignitability, a container is considered "RCRA-empty" if all the contents have been removed that can be removed by common means *and* no more than 3% remains (U.S. EPA, 2010b). For example, if the contents of an IV bag have been fully administered but droplets of the regulated drug remain in the IV tubing, this would meet the definition of RCRA empty, and the entire set could be disposed as trace chemotherapy rather than hazardous waste. Practically, then, if any HD remains in an IV bag, vial, or syringe, it is *not* "RCRA-empty" and should be discarded as hazardous waste. Items including needles, syringes, empty drug vials, ampoules, IV tubing, IV bags or bottles, and connecting devices should be discarded in the yellow trace-chemotherapy container to ensure disposal by incineration and to protect HCWs, including environmental services personnel, from exposure. Such items should be discarded intact to reduce the possibility of dispersing drug droplets. For this and other reasons, crushing or clipping needles is not recommended (OSHA, 1995). These containers must be puncture-proof so that they can safely sequester needles and other sharps. Use of protected needle devices for intramuscular or subcutaneous injections of HDs is highly recommended. A disposal container should be present at the site of drug administration to eliminate the need to transport an exposed needle. This recommendation also applies when discontinuing an IV access device with an exposed needle. Soft trace-contaminated items, such as gauze, wipes, and paper drapes, can be placed into either the yellow sharps containers or into yellow hamper bags labeled as "chemotherapy waste" and also incinerated as regulated medical waste.

PPE, such as gowns, gloves, or face shields, worn during drug handling should be disposed of in either the yellow trace-chemotherapy container or the yellow hamper bag. Reusable items that have been contaminated should be handled while wearing PPE and cleansed with soap and water before being returned to use. Disposable items contaminated by body fluids of patients who have received HDs in the previous 48 hours are considered contaminated. Discard disposable items such as pads, diapers, urinals, bedpans, measuring devices, Foley catheters, and drainage bags in the trace-chemotherapy container. Drainage collected following an HD bladder instillation should also be disposed in the trace-chemotherapy container. Because the returned drug is "used as intended," it is no longer regulated under RCRA, and it is biohazardous, which is appropriate for the trace-chemotherapy waste stream.

Avoid overfilling disposal containers. HCWs should not reach into hazardous waste containers when discarding contact material. Seal waste containers when three-fourths full. Once they are sealed, notify the appropriate personnel to remove the waste containers from the preparation or administration area. Only individuals who wear appropriate PPE and who have been trained regarding the exposure risks should handle the hazardous waste containers.

Hazardous pharmaceutical wastes should be managed separately from other hospital trash. Hazardous waste must be stored in a secure storage accumulation area in covered, leakproof containers or drums with distinct labels including the words *hazardous waste*. Additional labeling, manifesting, and other paperwork must be generated prior to shipping by a hazardous waste vendor who meets all EPA, Department of Transportation, and state requirements. Cradle-to-grave tracking is required, and the hospital retains full liability for ensuring proper disposal and documentation. The safety officer, facility manager, or environmental services manager is normally responsible for these activities. HD waste must be incinerated at a federally permitted treatment, storage, and disposal facility. All those involved in HD disposal must maintain records related to its transport and disposal. Yellow trace-chemotherapy waste should be stored with other regulated medical waste and be incinerated at a regulated medical waste facility, not autoclaved.

Management of Spills

Appropriate equipment and techniques should always be used to prevent inadvertent HD spills (see Table 8). However, despite precautions, environmental contamination can still occur. Large spills present a greater hazard potential and re-

Table 8. Techniques and Equipment for Spill Prevention

Potential Spill Situations	Preventive Interventions	Rationale
Reconstituting and preparing HD	Perform in PEC.	Minimizes escape of HD
	Consider CSTD.	Additional safety device
Spiking IV bags containing HD	Perform in PEC.	Minimizes escape of HD
	Add HD to IV bag after spiking.	Prevents leakage of HD
	Consider CSTD.	Additional safety device
Priming IV tubing	Prime tubing with nondrug solution.	Prevents dripping of HD from end of tubing
Leaking connections	Use locking connections.	Prevents disconnect associated with needles
	Consider CSTD.	Prevents flow of HD unless connected to Luer device
Inadvertent disconnect	Attach CSTD to distal end of tubing.	Prevents flow of HD unless connected to Luer device
Unspiking IV bag containing HD	Place HD on secondary set.	Allows tubing to be flushed with nondrug solution
	Discard tubing with IV bag attached instead of removing bag.	Removing bag can spread drops or result in aerosolization of HD.
Connecting/disconnecting IVP syringes	Attach CSTD to end of syringe.	Prevents leakage from syringe before administration and during disconnect
Purging air from syringes containing HD	Remove air bubbles inside PEC.	Prevents leakage from syringe, particularly if plunger sticks
Transporting leaking syringes or IV bags	Place all HDs in leakproof bags.	Bags will contain HD.
	Consider CSTD on syringe/IV bag.	Prevents leakage during transport
Excreta containing HD and metabolites	Use urinals with tight-fitting lids.	Prevents spilling of HD-containing urine
	Educate support staff regarding safe handling of excreta.	All staff should be aware of the potential for contamination and the need for PPE.
	Post signs for 48 hours after patient receives HDs.	

CSTD—closed-system drug transfer device; HD—hazardous drug; IV—intravenous; IVP—intravenous push; PEC—primary engineering control; PPE—personal protective equipment

---

quire more equipment for containment; however, even a small-volume spill of a volatile agent should be considered a source of exposure and handled appropriately. For this reason, spill kits must be available wherever HDs are stored, prepared, or administered.

Nurses who handle HDs should know where to access a spill kit, and designated employees who are responsible for managing HD spills must be properly trained (OSHA, 2004). Organizations may use a Hazardous Material Response Team for large-volume HD spills. Policies must clearly designate who is responsible for handling HD spills and outline the cleanup procedures.

Access to the area around an HD spill should be limited to personnel directly involved with cleanup operations, and patients should be moved away from the spill until it has been adequately cleaned. A sign should be posted to alert staff not involved in the cleanup, as well as patients and visitors.

Spill kits can be purchased commercially or assembled by the individual institution. Kits should minimally contain the items listed in Figure 11. All personnel involved with cleaning a spill are required to wear PPE, which includes a gown, double gloves, respiratory protection, and a face shield.

Deactivation

Conflicting evidence exists regarding the use of chemicals to deactivate HDs. Ideally, a product would be easy to use, work quickly, and be effective for all types of chemotherapy. Early studies demonstrated efficacy of calcium hypochlorite against several HDs in the laboratory (Dorr & Alberts, 1992). Sodium hypochlorite (bleach solution) has also been studied and shown to be effective against many but not all HDs (Benvenuto et al., 1993; Castegnaro et al., 1997; Roberts, Khammo, McDonnell, & Sewell, 2006). These studies were performed using a 5.25% concentration, which is equivalent to undiluted household bleach. However, this concentration creates potentially toxic fumes when used indoors to treat a spill, thereby limiting its application outside of the laboratory setting.

A less toxic product is commercially available. Surface Safe* contains two pads: one containing 2% sodium hypochlorite with detergent, and a second containing sodium thiosulfate (ASHP, 2006). The 2006 ASHP guidelines include its use for decontaminating PECs, but limited information exists regarding its efficacy for spills.

Detergent solutions are recommended for their ability to dilute, lift, and remove chemotherapy from a nonporous surface; however, it should be noted they do not inactivate or neutralize HDs. Other chemicals should not be used because toxic, unpredictable reactions may occur.

Figure 11. Hazardous Drug Spill Kit Contents

- Absorbent chemotherapy pads and towels
- 2 disposable chemotherapy-resistant gowns (with back closure)
- 2 pairs of chemotherapy-resistant shoe covers
- 4 pairs of chemotherapy gloves
- 2 pairs of chemical splash goggles
- 2 respirator masks approved by the National Institute for Occupational Safety and Health
- 1 disposable dustpan
- 1 plastic scraper
- 1 puncture-proof container for glass
- 2 large heavy-duty waste sealable disposal bags
- 1 hazardous waste label (if bags are unlabeled)

Note. Based on information from American Society of Health-System Pharmacists, 2006.

Procedure for Cleanup of Hazardous Drug Spills

- Assess the exposure of any individual involved, and isolate the individual from the spill.
- If the individual's clothing or skin has made contact with the hazardous agent, immediately remove the contaminated clothing and wash the skin with soap and water. (See Acute Exposure section for additional information.)
- Evacuate patients and personnel not involved in spill cleanup from the area.
- All individuals involved with the spill cleanup must don PPE, including double gloves, gown, and face shield.
- Wear a NIOSH-approved respirator. Standard paper surgical masks are ineffective. Note that N95 and N100 respirators are indicated for particles such as those generated by powders or aerosolization (spray). If the spilled chemotherapy is in liquid form, only canister-type respirators are indicated for vapors. Consult the MSDS of the spilled HD to determine the most appropriate respirator.
- Contain the spill using absorbent spill-control pads or towels.
- If possible, obtain assistance from another person who can hold the spill waste disposal bag. This will prevent contamination of the bag when discarding absorbent pads and other materials inside.
- Place pads or towels into the waste disposal bag, avoiding contamination of the mouth of the bag.
- Spills originating from chest or waist height can cause droplets to spread several feet from the source. HCWs need to evaluate the extent of these droplets by moving away from the spill and checking under patient beds, carts, and tables while using a good light source in order to ensure the entire spill is cleaned.
- Avoid touching any other parts of the environment during spill cleanup because gloves will most likely be contaminated.
- Use a detergent solution or Surface Safe* and detergent combination to clean the spill three times, beginning with the least contaminated area and finishing with

*See Clinical Update on page viii.

the most contaminated area. This prevents spreading of the spilled drug to less contaminated areas.

- Rinse area with plain water. Adequate dilution of HD residue is necessary to ensure that drug and any chemical residue has been removed and transferred to the wipes.
- Carefully remove PPE. Start with the outer gloves, then gown, then inner gloves, and discard in the waste bag, avoiding contamination of the bag. Seal the waste bag and place it in a puncture-proof container designated for HD waste. Wash hands thoroughly with soap and water.
- Clean reusable items contaminated by HDs following the previous steps. Wear PPE during cleaning, and dispose of it appropriately.

For Broken Glass

Pick up glass fragments by using a small scoop or by donning utility gloves over chemotherapy gloves. Place glass in the puncture-proof container using the designated scoop. Discard the scoop with other cleanup materials.

Spills on Carpeting

To clean an HD spill on a carpeted area, don PPE, including a respirator mask. Use an absorbent powder such as Green Z™ (Safetec of America, Inc.) to absorb the spill. Use a small vacuum cleaner dedicated for this purpose to remove the dried powder. Clean the carpet according to the institutional procedure. Little literature addresses HD spills on carpeting. Prudent practice suggests that a vacuum used in spill cleanup should be equipped with a HEPA filter to contain the HD-contaminated absorbent powder and limit further environmental contamination.

Spills Within a Biologic Safety Cabinet

ASHP recommends the use of a spill kit if the volume of the spill within a BSC or other PEC exceeds 30 ml or the contents of one drug vial (ASHP, 2006). Use utility gloves to remove any broken glass and place in a puncture-resistant HD container inside of a PEC. Clean and decontaminate the BSC using sodium hypochlorite solution or Surface Safe*, followed by a sterile water rinse, and then alcohol. If the spill contaminates the HEPA filter, the PEC should be sealed with plastic and not used until the filter can be replaced (ASHP, 2006).

For all spills, complete an incident or variance report to document occurrence. Include events leading up to the spill, the drug involved, the estimated volume of the spill, the cleanup procedures used, any individuals exposed, and those directly involved with the cleanup. Exposed individuals should be referred for medical evaluation, as described later in the Follow-Up section.

Hazardous Drug Spills at Home

The growing use of home infusion chemotherapy also increases the likelihood of a spill occurring outside of the hospital or clinic setting. Nurses working in the homecare setting must be trained in proper safe handling techniques and be able to provide patient education. Patients should be given a prepackaged spill kit with easy-to-follow instructions on how to clean themselves and their environment, how to dispose of contaminated materials, and to whom they should report the spill (Polovich et al., 2009).

*See Clinical Update on page viii.

Acute Exposure

Even with the diligent use of PPE and meticulous attention to safe handling techniques, accidental exposures to HDs can occur. Exposure can involve contamination of clothing, protective equipment, skin, mucous membranes, or the respiratory tract. HCWs may also be unknowingly exposed (Ben-Ami, Shaham, Rabin, Melzer, & Ribak, 2001; Labuhn, Valanis, Schoeny, Loveday, & Vollmer, 1998). In clinical practice, many accidental exposures may go unnoticed or unreported. It is imperative that nurses be attentive to the possibility of exposure.

The following steps should be taken in the event of a known exposure (ASHP, 2006).

- Immediately remove PPE and clothing that has been contaminated, taking care not to spread the contamination.
- Wash affected areas immediately with soap and water. Although evidence shows that dermal absorption is a significant concern, no specific recommendations exist for how long the skin should be cleansed.
- If eyes are affected, rinse for 15 minutes with water or an isotonic eyewash. If an eyewash station is not available, this can be accomplished by connecting IV tubing to a bag of 0.9% sodium chloride.
- The exposed individual should follow up with the employee health nurse for triage or go directly to the emergency room, as institutional policy directs.

Inhalation and Ingestion Exposure

Certain HDs have been shown to vaporize between 27°C and 37°C (80.6°F–98.6°F) (Connor et al., 2000). However, outside of the laboratory, little is known about the behavior of all HDs at various temperature and concentrations. Neither ASHP nor OSHA provides specific guidelines on the management of accidental inhalation of HDs in powdered form or procedures for accidental ingestion. The best resources for these types of exposure are MSDSs, which contain information on steps to take in the event of accidental exposure. MSDSs are provided by the drug company and also are available through other sources online. Each MSDS includes information on signs and symptoms of exposure, acute and chronic health hazards, and emergency or first-aid procedures.

In the event of accidental exposure, the exposed individual, or those treating the individual, should review applicable MSDSs. In some instances, the MSDS provides limited information and refers to the drug's package insert. MSDSs and package inserts should be available wherever HDs are prepared or administered or in a central location (e.g., pharmacy, emergency department, occupational health) where they can be accessed quickly. Additional advice may be obtained from the medical affairs department of the specific manufacturer.

Follow-Up

All employees exposed during spill cleanup should receive monitoring and follow-up care (ASHP, 2006). The medical care should be based on the exposure and may be different for various routes of exposure and types of HDs. This may occur in an employee health department, occupational health clinic, emergency department, or elsewhere as designated in institutional policies.

Accidental exposure can occur in any setting. Therefore, nurses working in inpatient areas, home care, outpatient clinics, and all other settings must possess the appropriate protocols for dealing with accidental HD exposure (ASHP, 2006; NIOSH, 2004).

Medical Surveillance of Healthcare Workers Handling Hazardous Drugs

Introduction

The inherent toxicity and mode of action of many anticancer agents combined with reports of therapy-related secondary malignancies in treated patients drove early efforts to minimize HD exposure in HCWs out of concern about cancer risk (Connor & McDiarmid, 2006). More recently, however, adverse reproductive health effects have surfaced as biologically plausible outcomes that have added new urgency to attempts at controlling workplace exposure. Nurses and pharmacists who are exposed to HDs in their workplaces have reported an increased number of adverse reproductive events, including spontaneous abortions, stillbirths, and congenital malformations, compared to unexposed HCWs (Hemminki, Kyyronen, & Lindbohm, 1985; Selevan, Lindbohm, Hornung, & Hemminki, 1985; Stücker et al., 1990; Valanis, Vollmer, & Steele, 1999). Importantly, recent studies have reported increases in miscarriages, preterm births, and infertility (Martin, 2005a), as well as increases in time to conception and low-birth-weight offspring (Fransman, Roeleveld, et al., 2007) as a function of exposure intensity. These reports and others highlight the health risks that HD handlers still face in the course of handling these agents (Eisenberg, 2009).

The classical occupational health approach to controlling exposure to workplace hazards by applying a combination of exposure control technologies also pertains to the healthcare venue. In addition to using engineering controls, safer work practices, and PPE to control and prevent exposure to HDs, workers who handle these agents should be routinely monitored in a medical surveillance program (ASHP, 2006; NIOSH, 2007; OSHA, 1995). Although NIOSH and ASHP have recently renewed calls for adoption of surveillance activity in comprehensive programs of exposure control, the recommendation for such inclusion is close to 20 years old (OSHA, 1995). Historical compliance with a surveillance provision has been poor, and recent surveys report only moderate compliance (Martin & Larson, 2003). This gap in adoption of recommendations for a comprehensive approach to manage workplace exposure is particularly troubling because it occurs in the absence of both specific federal regulations to protect exposed workers and recommended exposure levels to guide compliance (Gambrell & Moore, 2006).

What Is Medical Surveillance?

Medical surveillance involves the collection and interpretation of data for the purpose of detecting changes in the health status of working populations. Surveying the health status of a group of workers is a component of a comprehensive approach to hazard control. If exposure to a hazardous therapeutic drug or its aerosol cannot be eliminated through substitution of a less-dangerous agent or satisfactorily captured through engineering controls, then administrative controls and personal protective apparel (gloves, gowns, footwear protection) and equipment (respirators) are vital to minimize exposure (Niland, 1994). Medical surveillance is considered an administrative control in the hazard control hierarchy because it is a policy-oriented approach requiring an administrative decision by the employer to implement.

The general purpose of surveillance is to minimize adverse health effects in personnel exposed to potentially hazardous agents (Baker, Honchar, & Fine, 1989; McDiarmid & Emmett, 1987; Wesdock & Sokas, 2000). Surveillance is longitudinal in scope and geared to follow employees over their working lifetime. Medical surveillance programs involve assessment and documentation of symptom complaints, physical findings, and laboratory values (such as a blood count) to determine whether there is a deviation from the expected norms.

Medical surveillance can also be viewed as a secondary prevention tool providing a means of early detection of a health problem. Tracking employees through medical surveillance allows the comparison of health variables over time in individual workers, which may facilitate early detection of a change in a laboratory value or health condition. Medical surveillance programs also look for trends in populations of workers. Examining grouped data and comparing it to data from unexposed workers may reveal a small alteration or increase in the frequency of disease that would be obscured if individual workers' results alone were considered.

The work environment also can undergo surveillance. This usually involves an inspection for hazards, as well as air or work surface monitoring for the presence of hazardous contaminants. Surveillance, both medical and environmental, complements the use of engineering controls and good work practices, providing feedback on their efficacy. This feedback can be an impetus for the implementation of alternative or additional measures to minimize exposures and prevent adverse outcomes.

Elements of Medical Surveillance

Any medical surveillance program contains four data-gathering elements: history (medical and occupational), physical examination, laboratory studies, and biologic monitoring. Taken together, these elements give a reasonably comprehensive view of the health status of a worker and of a population of workers. Each component of medical surveillance helps to track the progression of workplace exposure from initial contact with HDs through ultimate biologic effects (see Figure 12).

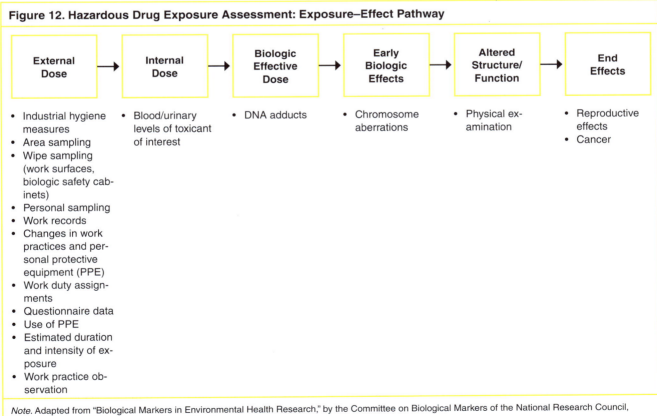

Figure 12. Hazardous Drug Exposure Assessment: Exposure–Effect Pathway

Note. Adapted from "Biological Markers in Environmental Health Research," by the Committee on Biological Markers of the National Research Council, 1987, Environmental Health Perspectives, 74, p. 4.

The exposure history elements of a surveillance program facilitate the identification of employees who are potentially at increased risk for adverse health events and provide a semi-quantitative estimate of external dose (e.g., duration of drug handling and administration). Information on exposure levels (i.e., intensity) in work areas, employee duty assignments, and questionnaires that assess the frequency of drug handling can help to estimate the external dose to which an employee has been exposed. The physical examination may yield signs of early biologic effects from exposure to HDs (i.e., skin lesions and hair loss) (Rogers & Emmett, 1987). Results from laboratory studies and biologic monitoring can help to quantify the internal dose of HDs. Biologic monitoring can potentially indicate exposure to a biologically effective dose or evidence of genotoxicity. The results of these studies give both direct and indirect evidence of an employee's exposure and the adverse health outcomes that may result. Ideally, medical surveillance can determine whether HCWs who are exposed to HDs are at risk for adverse health outcomes before they occur (by picking up early signs of exposure) and provide the opportunity for early intervention.

Targeted medical surveillance for HD handlers may be incorporated into ongoing employee health evaluations. Preplacement histories and medical examinations are important components of medical surveillance to document each worker's baseline health status. In addition, it is important to perform periodic examinations that gather the same information about signs, symptoms, and laboratory measures over time so that workers are monitored throughout their employment and any changes in health status can be assessed.

History

A thorough history is probably the best and most cost-effective source of useful health information. Medical and occupational information is obtained via questionnaire. Questionnaires are an efficient means of collecting a standardized set of information and provide documentation of changes in symptoms or the onset of health problems over time. The questionnaire should be reviewed with the worker to clarify answers and obtain more detail for responses that suggest a potential health effect.

Medical history: The medical history helps clinicians to interpret laboratory data obtained in the surveillance program, or it may identify a worker at potentially high risk in a particular exposure setting. For example, a person with documented asthma is at increased risk in a job where exposure to respiratory irritants or sensitizers is possible. Symptoms discovered in the medical history may serve as an early warning of a potential problem (i.e., sentinel health event) to the healthcare professional. Symptom questions should focus on organ systems that are targets for the hazardous agent or agents in question. The preplacement medical history should be very detailed. Periodic evaluations can be less exhaustive, focusing on signs and symptoms related to HD exposure and changes in health status since the previous evaluation.

Recording symptoms thought to be caused by HD exposure may give insight into drug-handling practices and alert health professionals to a potential problem. For example, complaints of light-headedness and dizziness were reported in antineoplastic drug handlers who did not use recommended handling procedures (Crudi, 1980; Ladik, Stoehr, & Maurer, 1980). In addition, a group of nurses exposed to HDs had significantly more hair loss and headaches than did unexposed controls (Rogers & Emmett, 1987). These symptoms and others known to occur in HD-treated patients should be investigated when reported by exposed HCWs. Further symptom questions should focus on the known target organs of the agent of exposure. In the case of antineoplastic drugs, special emphasis should be given to the skin and the hematopoietic, hepatic, reproductive, and urinary systems. Constitutional symptoms, including significant unintentional weight loss, fever, malaise, and unexplained fatigue, may be associated with anemia and hematologic malignancies (Appelbaum, 2000; Shipp & Harris, 2000). These constitutional symptoms should be included in a checklist and pursued in greater detail if they are present. Changes in the presence or frequency of symptoms over time can be an important clue to health changes.

Special consideration should be given to the reproductive history of employees handling HDs. General questions regarding problems in conceiving and poor reproductive outcomes (spontaneous abortions and congenital malformations) should be included. Male employees should provide information about the reproductive histories of their partners. For female employees, it is useful to request a complete reproductive history of each pregnancy, including dates, outcome, and work history during pregnancy. A sample medical history questionnaire is shown in Figure 13.

Work history: Estimating drug-handling history serves as a surrogate measure of the potential exposure dose. Knowing whether drug handlers wear PPE, such as gowns, gloves, face shields, or eye protection, will assist healthcare professionals in determining the opportunity for exposure. Use of a BSC during preparation of HDs also should be noted. Documentation of past untoward events, such as accidents and spills, assists occupational health professionals in estimating opportunity for exposure. A review of the frequency and duration of HD handling can be included in the periodic medical examination.

Physical Examination

The physical examination is probably the least helpful source of surveillance data, given the disease outcomes of concern in potentially exposed workers. However, a baseline examination is useful for documentation of any preexisting findings. Periodic examinations should focus on the skin and mucous membranes. The clinician should look for signs of rash, irritation, or other evidence of acute exposure. Evaluation of other target organ systems is also desirable. For example, hepatomegaly, splenomegaly, and lymph node enlargement may be associated with hematologic malignancies (Appelbaum, 2000; Shipp & Harris, 2000). In general, the hematopoietic, hepatic, renal, and urinary systems are more easily evaluated with laboratory studies, and significant illness is likely to be identified from the medical history and symptom queries.

Laboratory Studies

A tiered approach is helpful in selecting laboratory studies to include in a surveillance battery. In the first tier, studies that are desirable, at least as a baseline measure, should include a complete blood count with differential to monitor hematopoietic function (NIOSH, 2007). A urine dipstick test or a microscopic examination of the urine for blood may be helpful because some HDs cause bladder damage and hematuria in treated patients (Cronin & Henrich, 2000). Second-tier measures that are less crucial may include a reticulocyte count as an indication of bone marrow reserve. To follow hepatic function, liver transaminase concentrations (e.g., aspartate transaminase, alanine aminotransferase) and alkaline phosphatase may be measured. Altered liver function test results and evidence of liver damage have been reported in nurses handling antineoplastic drugs (Sotaniemi et al.,

PAGE 62 SAFE HANDLING OF HAZARDOUS DRUGS, SECOND EDITION

Figure 13. Sample Medical History Questionnaire for Hazardous Drug Handlers

A. Medical History

1. In the course of the past year, have you had any changes in your general health?

     _____ YES _____ NO

   If yes, please describe: _____

   _____

2. In the course of the past year, have you had any of the following symptoms?

	Yes	No	Have you noticed that these symptoms occur in relation to your work (e.g., either during the workday or immediately after)?
Bruising			
Dizziness			
Facial flushing			
Fever			
Gastrointestinal complaints			
Hair loss			
Headache			
Nausea			
Nosebleed			
Respiratory symptoms			
Skin rash			
Sore throat			
Vomiting			
Wheezing			
Other (Specify):			

   Unintentional weight loss ___ YES ___ NO   If yes, how many pounds? _____

3. In the course of the past year, or since you last completed this questionnaire, have you had any of the following **reproductive events** listed below?

   a) Have you or your partner ever had a problem conceiving a child? _____ YES _____ NO

   b) Have you or your partner consulted a physician for a fertility or other reproductive problem? _____ YES _____ NO

      If yes, who consulted the physician? ___ self ___ partner ___ self and partner

      If yes, please state the diagnosis that was made: _____

   c) In the past year, have you or your partner conceived a child resulting in a miscarriage, stillbirth, or birth defect?
      _____ YES _____ NO

      If yes, please specify the type of outcome: _____ Miscarriage _____ Stillbirth _____ Birth defect

      If the outcome was a birth defect, please specify the type or describe: _____

      _____

   d) What is the occupation of your spouse or partner? _____

   e) For women only: In the past year, have you had any menstrual irregularities? _____ YES _____ NO

      If yes, please specify the type of menstrual irregularity: _____

      If yes, how many episodes of this irregularity did you have (in the past year)?_____

(Continued on next page)

SAFE HANDLING OF HAZARDOUS DRUGS, SECOND EDITION

Figure 13. Sample Medical History Questionnaire for Hazardous Drug Handlers (Continued)

B. Work History

1. How many hours a week do you usually work with hazardous drugs (either handling or in the area where they are being handled)? _____

2. Has this schedule changed over the past year? _____ YES _____ NO

   If yes, how has it changed? _____
   _____

3. In the course of the past year, have you been around an antineoplastic drug spill?_____ YES _____ NO

   If yes, please give approximate date or dates (if this occurred more than once)._____

   If yes, approximately how large was the spill? _____ Less than 5 ml _____ More than 5 ml

   If yes, did you clean it up? _____ YES _____ NO

   If yes, what protective clothing were you wearing when the spill occurred?_____
   _____

4. In the course of the past year, have you accidentally ingested, breathed in, or had skin contact with an antineoplastic drug or solution?_____ YES _____ NO

   If yes, how often? _____

5. Please check the most appropriate answer as it applies to your antineoplastic drug-handling practice:

	Always	Often	Sometimes	Rarely	Never
I wear disposable gloves.					
I wear double gloves.					
I change my gloves according to the guidelines on my unit.					
I wear disposable gowns.					
I wear eye protection (goggles).					
I wear a protective mask.					
I wear disposable booties.					
I wear disposable hair covers.					
If I mix drugs, I use a biologic safety cabinet.					

Note. Based on information from McDiarmid & Curbow, 1992.

1983). Although several antineoplastic agents (e.g., cisplatin) have toxic effects on the kidney in patients receiving therapeutic doses (Cronin & Henrich, 2000), little renal toxicity has been documented to date in HD handlers. The usefulness of serum creatinine to assess renal toxicity is therefore uncertain for these workers. Figure 14 provides a list of the suggested laboratory studies. These tests are relatively inexpensive, and any that are not already part of an employee health evaluation program can be added to a routine panel that may already be in place. The frequency of periodic surveillance can be flexible, does not necessarily need to occur annually, and can be integrated into other existing surveillance schedules.

Biologic Monitoring

Biologic monitoring is the measurement of a specific agent or its metabolite in the body fluid of an exposed

---

Figure 14. Suggested Laboratory Tests for Medical Surveillance of Hazardous Drug Handlers

Tier 1*
- Complete blood count
- Urine microscopy or dipstick for blood

Tier 2**
- Reticulocyte count
- Liver transaminases (aspartate transaminase, alanine aminotransferase)
- Alkaline phosphatase

* Desirable; ** Optional

worker (Lauwerys, 1984; McDiarmid & Curbow, 1992). With the exception of following a worker subsequent to a major spill, the value of performing biologic monitoring for a specific drug is limited because workers who handle HDs may be exposed to multiple agents. This makes it difficult to choose which agent or agents to monitor. It is not feasible to perform such monitoring on all employees for the many agents in regular use.

Difficulties in the interpretation of mutagenicity measures and cytogenetic end points are a major limitation to their inclusion in routine medical surveillance. It is not possible to offer an accurate interpretation of an individual's positive urine mutagenicity test or to predict disease development for most cytogenetic outcomes, nor is it possible to definitely link any single positive result to occupational exposure. A positive result may provoke unnecessary anxiety in individuals for whom its importance cannot be adequately explained. Until more clarification of the clinical implications of these test results is available, biologic monitoring for genotoxic outcomes is not a recommended component of routine medical surveillance for HD handlers.

Acute Exposure Follow-Up

For acute exposure, such as after a spill on the skin or mucous membranes, the worker should have a postexposure evaluation. This evaluation is tailored to the type of exposure (e.g., spills or needlesticks). An assessment of the extent of exposure is made and included in an incident report or report of employee injury. The physical examination focuses on the involved area as well as other organ systems commonly affected (e.g., the skin and mucous membranes; the pulmonary system for aerosolized HDs). Treatment and laboratory studies follow as indicated and should be guided by emergency protocols. The occupational health professional should evaluate the need for specific follow-up based on the known toxicity of the agent in question and consult the MSDS.

The following are general suggestions for acute exposure management.
- Remove contaminated clothes, stockings, etc.
- Perform decontamination based on the MSDS for the agent of exposure.
- Visit the employee health professional to document and ensure complete decontamination.
- Perform a physical examination for acute findings at the site of exposure (e.g., skin or inhalation). Other aspects of the examination focus on target organs for the drug or drugs involved.
- Obtain blood for baseline counts and archiving (spin and freeze) so that there is something to compare in case of any excursion of outcomes. When collected immediately after an exposure, laboratory findings are almost as good as a preexposure draw.
- The employee health professional can determine appropriate follow-up times based on drug half-life and, for example, expected nadir of counts.
- Counseling should be provided to the individual as appropriate to the situation and may include waiting several (typically three) months before trying to conceive, what symptoms to report, and recommended medical follow-up.

Record Keeping

In addition to the periodic review of individual and grouped data to detect trends over time, OSHA (1995) recommends that an ongoing registry be maintained of all employees who routinely handle HDs. In the same way that a record is kept of the lifetime dose of certain chemotherapy drugs received by a patient, a drug-handling history should be maintained in the worker's employee health record. It is not necessary to record every instance of drug preparation and administration, although that would be ideal. This record should at least track the HCW by duration of assignment to an HD-handling job and the historical use of BSCs, safe work practices, and PPE. The drug-handling history then is used as a surrogate for exposure dose although "drug dose handled" and "exposure dose to the worker" are obviously not equivalent. The record can, however, be used to estimate the exposure dose and duration and may help in the interpretation of medical surveillance results.

The resources of an individual hospital or health system best determine the mechanics of a record-keeping program. The increasing use of computerized data systems to organize medical information provides the opportunity to incorporate records of occupational drug handling into the current databases.

Pharmacies typically keep a log to record each drug prepared and the name of the preparer. Pharmacies that issue computerized labels for each drug prepared may be able to modify their systems to internally record an identifier for the drug preparer. They also may generate several drug labels, which could be used in tracking the nurses who administer the drug. One label could be placed in the patient's chart and initialed by the nurse who gives the drug, and another label could be placed in an HD logbook and initialed by the nurse. The pharmacy preparation log and administration log could be reviewed periodically to compile a drug-handling history for each employee (McDiarmid, 1990). Electronic pharmacy systems that use bar codes to track drug preparation and administration may use electronic identification numbers to track personnel, which is another potentially useful means of estimating HD exposure for HCWs.

The employee health service and the safety committee should assist in implementing a record-keeping program to track employees who handle HDs. Data extraction from computerized information systems could result in automatic updates of exposure duration and intensity once the procedures are in place. These records would provide guidance in the interpretation of results from periodic medical surveillance of exposed employees.

Essential Components for Medical Surveillance of Hazardous Drug Handlers

Limited resources may preclude the implementation of a comprehensive medical surveillance program for HCWs who handle HDs. For institutions that do not have the means to develop a comprehensive surveillance program, a few key elements may serve to track employees' exposures (McDiarmid & Curbow, 1992). In healthcare institutions where some form of periodic employee health evaluation is already in place, new elements of surveillance may be added to screen HD handlers for their specific health risks.

- Maintain a list of all workers who are exposed to HDs as a part of their job.
- Have all HD handlers complete periodic questionnaires to track the frequency and duration of contact with these agents, their use of PPE, and any health events that are potentially related to HD exposure.
- Conduct periodic observations of drug preparation and administration practices to determine the need for refresher training in work practices that reduce exposure.
- Carefully document spills, spill cleanup activities, and accidental exposure.
- Confidentially share the results of medical surveillance with the employees who handle HDs.

- Settings without employee health professionals should develop policies that provide guidance for employees to pursue surveillance through their primary care providers.

Conclusions

A number of OSHA standards affecting the healthcare industry have medical surveillance provisions, including standards related to ethylene oxide, formaldehyde, and blood-borne pathogens. Therefore, including medical surveillance in a comprehensive approach to controlling adverse health outcomes from HD exposures in the healthcare setting is not novel. Tailoring of existing preplacement or periodic health evaluations performed at many institutions can integrate HD surveillance into an existing employee health program. When adverse outcomes are detected through medical surveillance, appropriate preventive actions should be taken to address any existing hazard. Engaged HCWs and employers, working in concert with employee health professionals, can successfully develop and implement a surveillance program that enhances health protection and promotes a work environment where these useful therapeutic agents are safely handled.

Staff Education and Training

Introduction

All nurses who handle HDs must be fully informed about the risks of exposure and about the strategies to mitigate those risks. But knowledge about safe handling precautions may not be enough to ensure compliance. Although nurses may know and understand the recommendations for safe handling, compliance with safe handling precautions varies (Eisenberg, 2009). Strategies designed to change attitudes and beliefs, in addition to enhancing knowledge and verifying skills, may be required to motivate the behavioral change necessary to increase compliance with recommendations and guidelines.

Although considerable information about safe handling practices has been disseminated, actual practice continues to lag behind published recommendations (McDiarmid & Condon, 2005; Valanis, McNeil, & Driscoll, 1991; Valanis, Vollmer, Labuhn, Glass, & Corelle, 1992). Use of PPE for HD administration tends to be lower than for equipment disposal and spill management (Mahon et al., 1994; Polovich, 2010). The available research suggests that nurses who handle HDs do not always adhere to recommended practices (Ben-Ami et al., 2001). In one survey, most participants (94%) indicated that they wore gloves when handling chemotherapy, but 55% wore laboratory coats rather than chemotherapy-designated gowns (Martin & Larson, 2003). Nieweg et al. (1994) reported similar findings in that most nurses wore gloves (91%) but far fewer (21%) wore gowns, and respondents reported deviations from recommended work practices.

Overall, a paucity of research exists about the factors influencing the use of HD safe handling precautions. Verity, Wiseman, Ream, Teasdale, and Richardson (2008) reported that British nurses often lacked confidence in their knowledge and skills when they initially administered chemotherapy, and they also reported considerable variation in preparation for this role. Most of the nurses in the study reported that they worried about their risk of exposure when handling these drugs. Based on interest expressed in educational programming about safe handling, it can be assumed that this is a topic of interest to nurses, but more research is needed to explore effective strategies for increasing the use of precautions. Polovich (2010) found that barriers such as the availability of PPE and their inconvenience interfered with precaution use.

Data exist that support the protection provided by PPE (Undeger, Basaran, Kars, & Guc, 1999; Ziegler, Mason, & Baxter, 2002), offering evidence that the use of gowns and gloves reduces HD exposure. In addition, a recent study of Indian nurses who administered HDs but did not use PPE reported genotoxicity in the nurses as measured by the comet assay (Rekhadevi et al., 2007). A pooled analysis of several studies in the Netherlands from 1997, 2000, and 2002 suggested that good work practices (such as use of locking connections and pre-priming tubing with saline) and an increased awareness of guidelines resulted in reduced HD exposure among nurses (Fransman, Peelen, et al., 2007). These findings indicate that education and training are necessary components of an HD safe handling program.

Most oncology nurses are knowledgeable about chemotherapy exposure and safe handling precautions (Polovich, 2010), but some clinicians do not perceive that they are personally vulnerable to health risks (e.g., "I have been doing this for years without wearing a gown and I am fine," or "I am beyond the childbearing years") (Martin, 2006). For example, nurses might choose to wear a laboratory coat instead of a chemotherapy-designated gown. These findings indicate that knowledge alone is insufficient to influence HD precaution use. Safe handling education must be designed to affect not only knowledge but also skills and attitudes.

Initial Education and Training

All HCWs who may be exposed to HDs—such as nurses and assistive personnel, physicians, pharmacists, housekeepers, and employees involved in receiving, transport, or storage—should participate in education and training specific to their role and job requirements prior to handling HDs.

Beyond oncology nurses and pharmacy personnel, workers who come in contact with HDs both in hospitals and other settings include
- Nursing assistants and patient care technicians who care for or handle the excreta of patients receiving HDs
- Nurses who work in areas such as rheumatology, the emergency department, and maternal-child areas and other non-oncology nurses who administer HDs
- Homecare nurses, nursing assistants, and formal and informal caregivers
- Transport personnel who deliver HDs from pharmacy preparation areas
- Transport personnel who move hazardous waste from satellite sites in patient care areas to storage areas
- Operating room or radiation therapy staff
- Environmental staff who clean patient rooms or administration areas
- Environmental staff who are tasked with spill response and cleanup
- Workers who receive and process HD shipments
- Nursing home workers
- Veterinary workers
- Laundry personnel.

All staff potentially at risk for HD exposure should be identified and included in systematic training programs (ASHP, 2006). Any worker expected to contain and decontaminate following an HD spill must receive comprehensive training on spill cleanup and the use of PPE and NIOSH-approved respirators. OSHA (1995) recommends that HD training be provided when an employee is first assigned to a work area where HDs are present and then annually, or more frequently if required, such as after a spill or other incident. Educational content should reflect institutional policies and be tailored for specific roles and job requirements.

Initial training and education should address some or all of the following elements, depending on job responsibilities.

- Potential health effects of HD exposure
  - Genotoxicity
  - Reproductive toxicity
  - Carcinogenicity
- Routes of occupational HD exposure
  - Dermal absorption
  - Ingestion
  - Inhalation
  - Injection
- PPE
  - Glove selection and use
  - Gown selection and use
  - Face and eye protection
  - Respiratory protection
  - Other equipment, such as shoe covers, for spill cleanup
- Engineering controls
  - BSCs or isolators
    * Proper installation and location
    * Maintenance and usage
  - CSTDs if available
- Work practice controls
  - Use of PPE
  - Appropriate removal and disposal of PPE
  - Drug storage practices
  - Drug preparation techniques that minimize exposure
    * Centralized drug preparation areas
    * Location of drug preparation area
    * Staff assignment for drug preparation
    * Gloves changed at appropriate intervals and when contaminated
    * Wiping down drug containers to remove drug residue
    * Hand-washing
    * Wiping down surfaces within the PEC
    * Appropriate disposal techniques
    * Priming all tubing with nondrug solution before adding HDs
    * Selection of the correct size of syringe to avoid overfilling
    * Capping syringes and transporting them without needles
    * Labeling of HDs with warning labels
  - Drug transport techniques to limit exposure
    * Use of containment devices, including placing in a clear, sealable plastic bag
    * Drug transportation process
  - Drug administration techniques to limit exposure
    * Use of locking connections
    * Use of CSTDs if available
    * Avoiding spiking and unspiking at the bedside or chairside
    * Using dry spiking and back-priming technique when needed
    * Wiping down the outside of drug containers
    * Considering the infusion tubing, connectors, and pumps available to determine the optimal technique for connecting IV HDs
    * Using plastic-backed absorbent pads to absorb leaks

- * Using gauze squares around injection ports or connections to absorb leaks
- * Avoiding ejecting air from syringes for intramuscular or subcutaneous injections outside the BSC
- * Managing skin, mucous membrane, or ocular contamination
- * Spill kit contents and use
- * Spill containment and management, including use of a respirator
  - Patient care
  - * Appropriate PPE
  - * Hand-washing
  - * Handling of contaminated fluids and excreta
  - * Cleaning of contaminated areas and equipment
  - * Handling linens
  - * Skin protection of the incontinent patient
  - * Safe handling issues in the home
- • Medical surveillance

Didactic content should be evaluated through some form of knowledge assessment, such as a quiz or test after a live educational program or following completion of a computer-based training program. In addition to knowledge assessment, competency for specific skills, such as spill cleanup, should be evaluated by direct observation. Fluorescent nondrug solutions, such as quinine (OSHA, 1995) or fluorescein (Dussart et al., 2008; Harrison, Godefroid, & Kavanaugh, 1996), can be used to evaluate drug-handling technique as the liquid will fluoresce under ultraviolet light, and any breaches in technique will be made obvious. A checklist, such as that found in Appendix A, provides one method of documenting competence in HD safe handling skills. Similar checklists reflecting institutional policies should be developed.

Periodic Education and Training

Each employee involved in HD handling should receive annual updates regarding new HDs, MSDSs, and HD policies, procedures, and other guidelines. Annual updates should review initial training, based on employee role, and should also include a review of PPE, medical surveillance if available, spill management, and acute exposure response. Training should include special attention to workers who do not speak English so that they recognize the warning signs and labels of HDs.

Special Educational Needs

Unique routes of administration, such as intravesical, IP, and intraoperative therapies, require that staff learn additional safe handling content (see Appendix B). Intravesical therapy using an indwelling catheter, for example, necessitates handling of a large volume of drainage from the bladder via a closed system (McDonald, 2007; Washburn, 2007), so appropriate containment equipment should be evaluated and made available. In all of these settings, safe handling procedures, adequate training, and supervised practice with necessary equipment should be provided prior to the initiation of treatments.

HDs administered in the home setting may pose additional challenges to ensuring that safe handling practices are implemented. Less control over the environment by professional staff with possible breaches in good practice can contribute to potential environmental contamination and other challenges (Meijster, Fransman, Veldhof, & Kromhout, 2006). Homecare programs should ensure that their nursing staff members receive adequate training in all aspects of

HD administration, patient care, safe handling, and patient and family education about safe handling practices.

Educational Strategies

Education and training designed to teach nurses and others about safe handling of HDs generally aims to augment knowledge about the potential hazards and how to avoid them, to develop specific psychomotor skills, and to engage in specific behaviors, such as the following.

- Work practice controls, such as wearing PPE and pre-priming IV bags with non-drug fluids, are taught as strategies to improve safe handling.
- Proper engineering controls, such as a BSC, isolator, or CSTDs, are used for drug preparation and administration.
- Administrative controls, such as requiring nurses to have an ONS Chemotherapy Provider Card and complete annual competency testing, also are recommended to make certain that nurses administering HDs are competent.

Some professional groups, such as those of nurses and pharmacists, have access to education and training developed by their professional organizations. Nurses who administer HDs perform their work in a variety of settings and with wide variation in their professional experience and specialized training. Many nurses participate in the ONS Chemotherapy and Biotherapy Course and receive a provider card following successful course completion (Polovich et al., 2009). Safe handling content is a component of the ONS course. As ONS guidelines recommend, nurses should complete a clinical practicum before administering chemotherapy (see Appendix B). As part of this component of their training, nurses should be precepted by experienced nurses in the actual administration of HDs and educated on the associated institutional policies. Provider card renewal requires additional periodic continuing education, thereby ensuring that knowledge will be updated and that the learner will review current trends and practices, including information about new therapies.

Adult Learning

Adult learning takes place across three domains as described in Bloom's taxonomy: knowledge (cognitive), psychomotor (skills and behaviors), and affective (attitudes) (Knowles, Holton, & Swanson, 2005). A clinical practicum blends all of these domains in the delivery of patient care. Programming on safe handling should address the requisite knowledge, skills, and attitudes to handle HDs safely and should incorporate the larger components of an organizational safety culture.

Learners use concrete experience, reflective observation, abstract conceptualization, and active experimentation as they attempt to integrate new learning (Kolb, 1984). For example, oncology nurses who have earned an ONS provider card return to their clinical setting and, through the clinical practicum or preceptor experience, engage in a variety of behaviors to continue their learning. As nurses learn to handle HDs safely, they gain insight from their new experience, make observations about their own practice and the practice of other nurses, conceptualize how they would handle a specific scenario (e.g., a drug spill), and then use their integrated knowledge to solve problems and make decisions in practice.

Effective continuing nursing education incorporates principles of adult learning in content delivery. Adults prefer self-directed educational experiences that are centered on action, based on their experience, focused on real-life problems, and driven by solutions. As adult learners, HCWs bring a wealth of personal and practical clinical experience to their professional practice. Respecting that expertise, drawing upon it, and building upon its foundation are important aspects of effective adult education. Creating connections between the material to be learned and content that the learner has already mastered is essential. In a culture where evidence-based practice is valued, highlighting new evidence can be an effective strategy to modify learner behavior.

Adults learn using different styles, and programming ideally should be offered in several formats to appeal to most learners. For some, visual presentations work best, so computer-based training or other visual strategies, such as reading a journal article or a self-study guide, might be the preferred learning mode. For those who are auditory learners, podcasts or recorded presentations might be used. Combined audiovisual presentations, such as recorded lectures with visuals, podcasts, or video programs, appeal to a wide range of learners. Distance-learning formats featuring computer-based training or blended formats allow learning to take place anywhere, at the time and setting of the learner's choice—a concept well suited to self-directed adult learners. Others learn best by doing, so experiential exercises, one-on-one coaching, and clinical practicums offer an ideal learning venue. Over time, comprehensive safe handling education can engage participants in discussion, journal clubs, reviews, practice-based scenarios, case studies, role play, and experiential exercises to keep the learning experience fresh and interesting.

Overcoming Barriers to Safe Handling Practices

Even the best teaching methodologies will fail to convince a certain segment of healthcare providers who feel that they are not susceptible to the adverse outcomes associated with handling HDs or who practice in a setting where the organizational culture minimizes the importance of safe handling recommendations. Eisenberg (2009, p. 28) summarizes many of the barriers to using PPE documented in the literature. These barriers include inconvenient access to equipment, inadequate supplies, gloves that do not fit or are difficult to put on, gowns that are uncomfortable, knowledge deficits, faulty belief systems, lack of time, psychological impact of PPE on patients, and habitual outdated practices.

Resistance to using PPE such as gowns with polyethylene or vinyl coating can be a barrier that affects staff behaviors and presents a challenge to training efforts. Valanis's early work in this area documented low levels of compliance with recommended safe handling precautions that were, in part, due to a lack of perceived susceptibility to harm (Valanis et al., 1991, 1992). Compliance with recommended practices evolves not only from knowledge but also from attitudinal beliefs and even peer pressure (Ben-Ami et al., 2001). Improvements in knowledge and skills, therefore, are insufficient to change the behavior of some nurses. Effective safe handling education should also seek to change attitudes and perceptions, targeting affective change in the learner as well as organizational culture in the work setting.

Educational strategies to address the affective domain of learning prove to be more elusive and may be neglected in the planning and execution of nursing education. Influencing attitudes is much more complex than changing behaviors or increasing knowledge. Long-standing beliefs (e.g., "I was pregnant while handling chemotherapy, and my child is fine," or "Patients will be frightened if I give their drugs dressed in a Hazmat suit") can be powerful forces in a clinical setting and may set the norms for accepted practice and safe handling behavior. Teaching strategies in this domain of learning assist the learner to internalize values and to demonstrate behaviors consistent with these values (e.g., "I will wear PPE consistently even if my coworkers do not").

Informal Education

Some HCWs benefit from formal continuing education or in-services, whereas others have learned about handling practices through on-the-job training or by self-study or consulting colleagues. Different settings of care may have varying practices, and staff members may have wide ranges of experience (Verity et al., 2008). As a result, informal on-the-job training may be inconsistent. Specialized centers may have more access to local expertise while some in lower-acuity settings may have fewer experienced staff members available or may lose staff with expertise by attrition.

Much of the knowledge transmitted in the clinical setting is conveyed from one practitioner to the next through conversation and dialogue, often occurring in the context of a preceptor or mentorship relationship. One example of informal learning is that of conversational learning, a process during which learners make sense of what they have learned and what they are experiencing through conversations (Baker, Jensen, & Kolb, 2002). Two individuals, such as a staff nurse and an advanced practice nurse, collaborate, and through the sharing of ideas and experiences, these professionally oriented conversations can be opportunities for learning. It is in these moments of informal teaching where the rationale for the use of PPE can be reinforced, or where the significance of specific work practice controls can be highlighted in the context of practice. What may have been unclear in the classroom or in front of a computer screen comes alive in the clinical setting under actual practice conditions.

Staff educated in safe handling should consistently role-model safe handling behaviors and compliance (Polovich, 2004). Role modeling of recommended practices by experienced and respected practitioners can go a long way in shaping the behaviors of new or less experienced staff. The converse is also true: the reluctance of more seasoned staff to change their practice to reflect current recommendations can be detrimental to the knowledge, practice, and attitudes of those they mentor. Informal educational interactions provide a perfect opportunity to stimulate a different perspective on these issues and to create an impetus for adapting recommended safe handling practices.

Innovative Strategies

Virtual patients, using strategies as diverse as written scenarios placed online to three-dimensional avatars (graphical images of people, such as those used in simulation computer games), are used in many clinical nursing education settings (Notarianni, Curry-Lourenco, Barham, & Palmer, 2009) and can provide opportunities to practice safe handling precautions. Another strategy, simulated practice, uses technologies such as high-fidelity simulators (Nehring & Lashley, 2010; Notarianni et al., 2009) and may be used in the continuing education of oncology nurses on safe handling precautions. Simulated practice has been used extensively in the teaching of cardiopulmonary resuscitation and holds promise as an oncology nursing education tool as well. Scenarios featuring a progressive simulation of a patient receiving chemotherapy and the care required to administer the chemotherapy could be created, such as using a CSTD, implementing recommended drug administration work practices, donning and removing PPE correctly, disposing of HD waste, handling patient excreta, cleaning up spills, and caring for patient in the home setting. Simulated safe handling learning situations allow learners to achieve learning goals without actual exposure to HDs.

In summary, all personnel who are responsible for any aspect of HD handling must be properly trained according to their specific role. While knowledge alone is insufficient to ensure HD safe handling, it is an essential component of an HD safe handling program.

References

Aiello-Laws, L., & Rutledge, D.N. (2008). Management of adult patients receiving intraventricular chemotherapy for the treatment of leptomeningeal metastasis. *Clinical Journal of Oncology Nursing, 12,* 429–435. doi:10.1188/08.CJON.429-435

American Cancer Society. (2009, October 7). Detailed guide: Penile cancer topical chemotherapy. Retrieved from http://www.cancer.org/Cancer/PenileCancer/DetailedGuide/penile-cancer-treating-chemotherapy

American Society of Health-System Pharmacists. (2006). ASHP guidelines on handling hazardous drugs. *American Journal of Health-System Pharmacy, 63,* 1172–1191.

American Society of Health-System Pharmacists. (2009). AHFS Drug Information®. Retrieved from http://online.statref.com

American Society of Health-System Pharmacists. (2010). AHFS Pharmacologic-Therapeutic Classification System. Retrieved from http://www.ahfsdruginformation.com/class/index.aspx

American Society of Hospital Pharmacists. (1990). ASHP technical assistance bulletin on handling cytotoxic and hazardous drugs. *American Journal of Hospital Pharmacy, 47,* 1033–1049.

American Society for Testing and Materials. (2005). *ASTM D6978-05: Standard practice for assessment of resistance of medical gloves to permeation by chemotherapy drugs.* West Conshohocken, PA: Author. doi:10.1520/D6978-05

Appelbaum, F.R. (2000). The acute leukemias. In L. Goldman & J.C. Bennett (Eds.), *Cecil textbook of medicine* (21st ed., pp. 953–958). Philadelphia, PA: Saunders.

Association for Linen Management. (2009). Proposed methodology for handling cytotoxic and other potentially hazardous drug contaminated linen safety and health plan for the institutional linen industry. Retrieved from http://www.almnet.org/displaycommon.cfm?an=15

Atmaca-Sonmez, P., Atmaca, L.S., & Aydintug, O.T. (2007). Update on ocular Behçet's disease. *Expert Review of Ophthalmology, 2,* 957–979. doi:10.1586/17469899.2.6.957

Baehring, J.M. (2008). Increased intracranial pressure. In V.T. DeVita Jr., T.S. Lawrence, & S.A. Rosenberg (Eds.), *Cancer: Principles and practice of oncology* (8th ed., Vol. 2, pp. 2435–2440). Philadelphia, PA: Lippincott Williams & Wilkins.

Baker, A., Jensen, P.J., & Kolb, D.A. (2002). *Conversational learning: An experiential approach to knowledge creation.* Westport, CT: Quorum Books.

Baker, E.L., Honchar, P.A., & Fine, L.J. (1989). Surveillance in occupational illness and injury: Concepts and content. *American Journal of Public Health, 79*(Suppl.), 9–11.

Baker, E.S., & Connor, T.H. (1996). Monitoring exposure to cancer chemotherapy drugs. *American Journal of Health-System Pharmacy, 53,* 2713–2723.

Bankhead, R., Boullata, J., Brantley, S., Corkins, M., Guenter, P., Krenitsky, J., ... A.S.P.E.N. Board of Directors. (2009). A.S.P.E.N. enteral nutrition practice recommendations. *Journal of Parenteral and Enteral Nutrition, 33,* 122–167. doi:10.1177/0148607108330314

Bartlett, D.L., Bisceglie, A.M., & Dawson, L.A. (2008). Cancer of the liver. In V.T. DeVita Jr., T.S. Lawrence, & S.A. Rosenberg (Eds.), *Cancer: Principles and practice of oncology* (8th ed., Vol. 1, pp. 1129–1155). Philadelphia, PA: Lippincott Williams & Wilkins.

Batchelor, T., & Supko, J.G. (2009). Experimental treatment approaches for malignant gliomas. Retrieved from http://www.uptodate.com

Ben-Ami, S., Shaham, J., Rabin, S., Melzer, A., & Ribak, J. (2001). The influence of nurses' knowledge, attitudes and health beliefs on their safe behavior with cytotoxic drugs in Israel. *Cancer Nursing, 24,* 192–200.

Benvenuto, J.A., Connor, T.H., Monteith, D.K., Laidlaw, J.L., Adams, S.C., Matney, T.S., & Theiss, J.C. (1993). Degradation and inactivation of antitumor drugs. *Journal of Pharmaceutical Sciences, 82,* 988–991.

Bertsias, G., Gordon, C., & Boumpas, D.T. (2008). Clinical trials in systemic lupus erythematosus (SLE): Lessons from the past as we proceed to the future—The EULAR recommendations for the management of SLE and the use of end-points in clinical trials. *Lupus, 17,* 437–442. doi:10.1177/0961203308090031

Bertsias, G.K., Ioannidis, J.P.A., Aringer, M., Bollen, E., Bombardieri, S., Bruce, I.N., ... Boumpas, D.T. (2010). EULAR recommendations for the management of systemic lupus erythematosus with neuropsychiatric manifestations: Report of a task force of the EULAR standing committee for clinical affairs. *Annals of the Rheumatic Diseases.* Advance online publication. doi:10.1136/ard.2010.130476

Brennan, M.F., Singer, S., Maki, R.G., & O'Sullivan, B. (2008). Soft tissue sarcoma. In V.T. DeVita Jr., T.S. Lawrence, & S.A. Rosenberg (Eds.), *Cancer: Principles and practice of oncology* (8th ed., Vol. 2, pp. 1741–1793). Philadelphia, PA: Lippincott Williams & Wilkins.

Brogan, P.A., & Dillon, M.J. (2000). The use of immunosuppressive and cytotoxic drugs in non-malignant disease. *Archives of Disease in Childhood, 83,* 259–264. doi:10.1136/adc.83.3.259

Brown, P.D., & Meyers, C.A. (2008). Neurocognitive effects. In V.T. DeVita Jr., T.S. Lawrence, & S.A. Rosenberg (Eds.), *Cancer: Principles and practice of oncology* (8th ed., Vol. 2, pp. 2751–2756). Philadelphia, PA: Lippincott Williams & Wilkins.

Burgaz, S., Karahalil, B., Canhi, Z., Terzioglu, F., Ançel, G., Anzion, R.B., ... Hüttner, E. (2002). Assessment of genotoxic damage in nurses occupationally exposed to antineoplastics by the analysis of chromosomal aberrations. *Human and Experimental Toxicology, 21,* 129–135.

Bussieres, J.F., Theoret, Y., Prot-Labarthe, S., & Larocque, D. (2007). Program to monitor surface contamination by methotrexate in a hematology-oncology satellite pharmacy. *American Journal of Health-System Pharmacy, 64,* 531–535.

Cannistra, S.A., Gershenson, D.M., & Recht, A. (2008). Ovarian cancer, fallopian tube carcinoma, and peritoneal carcinoma. In V.T. DeVita Jr., T.S. Lawrence, & S.A. Rosenberg (Eds.), *Cancer: Principles and practice of oncology* (8th ed., Vol. 2, pp. 1568–1594). Philadelphia, PA: Lippincott Williams & Wilkins.

Cantarini, M.V., McFarquhar, T., Smith, R.P., Bailey, C., & Marshall, A.L. (2004). Relative bioavailability and safety profile of gefitinib administered as a tablet or as a dispersion preparation via drink or nasogastric tube: Results of a randomized, open-label, three-period crossover study in healthy volunteers. *Clinical Therapeutics, 26,* 1630–1636. doi:10.1016/j.clinthera.2004.10.011

Castegnaro, M., De Méo, M., Laget, M., Michelon, J., Garren, L., Sportouch, M.H., & Hansel, S. (1997). Chemical degradation of wastes of antineoplastic agents. 2: Six anthracyclines: idarubicin, doxorubicin, epirubicin, pirarubicin, aclarubicin, and daunorubicin. *International Archives of Occupational and Environmental Health, 70,* 378–384. doi:10.1007/s004200050232

Cavallo, D., Ursini, C.L., Perniconi, B., Francesco, A.D., Giglio, M., Rubino, F.M., … Iavicoli, S. (2005). Evaluation of genotoxic effects induced by exposure to antineoplastic drugs in lymphocytes and exfoliated buccal cells of oncology nurses and pharmacy employees. *Mutation Research, 587,* 45–51. doi:10.1016/j.mrgentox.2005.07.008

Connor, T.H. (2005, November/December). External contamination of antineoplastic drug vials. *Hospital Pharmacy Europe,* Issue 23, 52–54. Retrieved from http://www.hospitalpharmacyeurope.com

Connor, T.H., Anderson, R.W., Sessink, P.J., Broadfield, L., & Power, L.A. (1999). Surface contamination with antineoplastic agents in six cancer treatment centers in Canada and the United States. *American Journal of Health-System Pharmacy, 56,* 1427–1432.

Connor, T.H., Anderson, R.W., Sessink, P.J., & Spivey, S.M. (2002). Effectiveness of a closed-system device in containing surface contamination with cyclophosphamide and ifosfamide in an I.V. admixture area. *American Journal of Health-System Pharmacy, 59,* 68–72.

Connor, T.H., & Eisenberg, S. (2010, May). *Safe handling of hazardous drugs: Risks and practical considerations.* Symposium presented at the Oncology Nursing Society 35th Annual Congress, San Diego, CA.

Connor, T.H., & McDiarmid, M.A. (2006). Preventing occupational exposures to antineoplastic drugs in health care settings. *CA: A Cancer Journal for Clinicians, 56,* 354–365. doi:10.3322/canjclin.56.6.354

Connor, T.H., Sessink, P.J., Harrison, B.R., Pretty, J.R., Peters, B.G., Alfaro, R.M., … Dechristoforo, R. (2005). Surface contamination of chemotherapy drug vials and evaluation of new vial-cleaning techniques: Results of three studies. *American Journal of Health-System Pharmacy, 62,* 475–484.

Connor, T.H., Shults, M., & Fraser, M.P. (2000). Determination of the vaporization of solutions of mutagenic antineoplastic agents at 23 and 37 degrees C using a desiccator technique. *Mutation Research, 470,* 85–92. doi:10.1016/S1383-5718(00)00105-4

Connor, T.H., & Xiang, Q. (2000). The effect of isopropyl alcohol on the permeation of gloves exposed to antineoplastic agents. *Journal of Oncology Pharmacy Practice, 6,* 109–114. doi:10.1177/107815520000600304

Controlled Environment Testing Association. (2007, January). CETA applications guide for the use of surface decontaminants in biosafety cabinets (CAG-004-2007; Adopted January 30, 2007). Retrieved from http://www.cetainternational.org/reference/CAG0042007i.pdf

Controlled Environment Testing Association. (2008). CETA applications guide for the use of compounding aseptic isolators in compounding sterile preparations in healthcare facilities (CAG-001-2005; Revised December 8, 2008). Retrieved from http://www.cetainternational.org/reference/ApplicationsGuideBarrierIsolator-CAG-001-2005.pdf

Cooke, J., Williams, J., Morgan, R.J., Cooke, P., & Calvert, R.T. (1991). Use of cytogenetic methods to determine mutagenic changes in the blood of pharmacy personnel and nurses who handle cytotoxic agents. *American Journal of Hospital Pharmacy, 48,* 1199–1205.

Cronin, R.E., & Henrich, W.L. (2000). Toxic nephropathies. In B.M. Brenner (Ed.), *Brenner and Rector's the kidney* (6th ed., pp. 1571–1573). St. Louis, MO: Saunders.

Crudi, C.B. (1980). A compounding dilemma: I've kept the drug sterile but have I contaminated myself? *Journal of Infusion Nursing, 3,* 77–78.

Dalakas, M.C. (2008). B cells as therapeutic targets in autoimmune neurological disorders. *Nature Clinical Practice Neurology, 4,* 557–567. doi:10.1038/ncpneuro0901

Dalakas, M.C. (2010a). Inflammatory muscle diseases: A critical review on pathogenesis and therapies. *Current Opinion in Pharmacology, 10,* 346–352. doi:10.1016/j.coph.2010.03.001

Dalakas, M.C. (2010b). Pathogenesis and treatment of anti-MAG neuropathy. *Current Treatment Options in Neurology, 12,* 71–83. doi:10.1007/s11940-010-0065-x

Dayton, C.S. (1996). Use of cytotoxic drug therapy in non-malignant pulmonary disease. *P&T News, 16*(7). Retrieved from http://www.healthcare.uiowa.edu/pharmacy/PTNews/1996/01.96.html

DeAngelis, L.M., & Yahalom, J. (2008). Primary central nervous system lymphoma. In V.T. DeVita Jr., T.S. Lawrence, & S.A. Rosenberg (Eds.), *Cancer: Principles and practice of oncology* (8th ed., Vol. 2, pp. 2159–2166). Philadelphia, PA: Lippincott Williams & Wilkins.

de Smet, M.D., Vancs, V.S., Kohler, D., Solomon, D., & Chan, C.C. (1999). Intravitreal chemotherapy for the treatment of recurrent intraocular lymphoma. *British Journal of Ophthalmology, 83,* 448–451. doi:10.1136/bjo.83.4.448

Deng, H., Zhang, M., He, J., Wu, W., Jin, L., Zheng, W., ... Wang, B. (2005). Investigating genetic damage in workers occupationally exposed to methotrexate using three genetic end-points. *Mutagenesis, 20,* 351–357. doi:10.1093/mutage/gei048

Dorr, R.T. (2001, May). *Achieving safe handling of cytotoxic agents: What is being done?* Paper presented at the 26th Annual Congress of the Oncology Nursing Society, San Diego, CA.

Dorr, R.T., & Alberts, D.S. (1992). Topical absorption and inactivation of cytotoxic anticancer agents in vitro. *Cancer, 70*(Suppl. 4), 983–987.

Driesen, P., Boutin, C., Viallat, J.R., Astoul, P.H., Vialette, J.P., & Pasquier, J. (1994). Implantable access system for prolonged intrapleural immunotherapy. *European Respiratory Journal, 7,* 1889–1892. doi:10.1183/09031936.94.07101889

Dussart, C., Favier, B., Gilles, L., Camal, I., Almeras, D., Latour, J.F., & Grelaud, G. (2008). [Continuous training program for technicians handling antineoplastic drugs and occupational exposure risk]. *Bulletin du Cancer, 95,* 821–822. doi:10.1684/bdc.2008.0706

Eisenberg, S. (2009). Safe handling and administration of antineoplastic chemotherapy. *Journal of Infusion Nursing, 32,* 23–32. doi:10.1097/NAN.0b013e31819246e0

Ellsworth-Wolk, J.M., & Maxson, J.H. (2005). Principles of preparation, administration, and disposal of hazardous drugs. In J.K. Itano & K.N. Taoka (Eds.), *Core curriculum for oncology nursing* (4th ed., pp. 802–808). Philadelphia, PA: Elsevier Saunders.

Favier, B., Gilles, L., Ardiet, C., & Latour, J.F. (2003). External contamination of vials containing cytotoxic agents supplied by pharmaceutical manufacturers. *Journal of Oncology Pharmacy Practice, 9,* 15–20. doi:10.1191/1078155203jp102oa

Favier, B., Rull, F.M., Bertucat, H., Pivot, C., LeBoucher, G., Charlety, D., ... Latour, J.F. (2001). Surface and human contamination with 5-fluorouracil in six hospital pharmacies. *Journal de Pharmacie Clinique, 20,* 157–162.

Foltz, P., Wavrin, C., & Sticca, R. (2004). Heated intraoperative intraperitoneal chemotherapy—The challenges of bringing chemotherapy into surgery. *AORN Journal, 80,* 1054–1063. doi:10.1016/S0001-2092(06)60684-4

Fox, R.I. (2000). Sjögren's syndrome: Current therapies remain inadequate for a common disease. *Expert Opinion on Investigational Drugs, 9,* 2007–2016. doi:10.1517/13543784.9.9.2007

Fransman, W., Huizer, D., Tuerk, J., & Kromhout, H. (2007). Inhalation and dermal exposure to eight antineoplastic drugs in an industrial laundry facility. *International Archives of Occupational and Environmental Health, 80,* 396–403. doi:10.1007/s00420-006-0148-x

Fransman, W., Peelen, S., Hilhorst, S., Roeleveld, N., Heederik, D., & Kromhout, H. (2007). A pooled analysis to study trends in exposure to antineoplastic drugs among nurses. *Annals of Occupational Hygiene, 51,* 231–239. doi:10.1093/annhyg/mel081

Fransman, W., Roeleveld, N., Peelen, S., de Kort, W., Kromhout, H., & Heederik, D. (2007). Nurses with dermal exposure to antineoplastic drugs: Reproductive outcomes. [Research]. *Epidemiology, 18,* 112–119.

Fransman, W., Vermeulen, R., & Kromhout, H. (2004). Occupational dermal exposure to cyclophosphamide in Dutch hospitals: A pilot study. *Annals of Occupational Hygiene, 48,* 237–244. doi:10.1093/annhyg/meh017

Fransman, W., Vermeulen, R., & Kromhout, H. (2005). Dermal exposure to cyclophosphamide in hospitals during preparation, nursing and cleaning activities. *International Archives of Occupational and Environmental Health, 78,* 403–412. doi:10.1007/s00420-004-0595-1

Fuchs, J., Hengstler, J.G., Jung, D., Hiltl, G., Konietzko, J., & Oesch, F. (1995). DNA damage in nurses handling antineoplastic agents. *Mutation Research, 342,* 17–23.

Gambrell, J., & Moore, S. (2006). Assessing workplace compliance with handling of antineoplastic agents. *Clinical Journal of Oncology Nursing, 10,* 473–477. doi:10.1188/06.CJON.473-477

Gangaputra, S., Nussenblatt, R., & Levy-Clarke, G. (2008). Therapeutic modalities for intraocular lymphoma. *Cancer Therapy, 6,* 131–136.

Garaj-Vrhovac, V., & Kopjar, N. (1998) Micronuclei in cytokinesis-blocked lymphocytes as an index of occupational exposure to antineoplastic drugs. *Radiotherapy and Oncology, 32,* 385–392.

Goloni-Bertollo, E.M., Tajara, E.H., Manzato, A.J., & Varella-Garcia, M. (1992). Sister chromatid exchanges and chromosome aberrations in lymphocytes of nurses handling antineoplastic drugs. *International Journal of Cancer, 50,* 341–344.

Gotlieb, W.H., Bruchim, I., Ben-Baruch, G., Davidson, B., Zeltser, A., Andersen, A., & Olsen, H. (2007). Doxorubicin levels in the serum and ascites of patients with ovarian cancer. *European Journal of Surgical Oncology, 33,* 213–215. doi:10.1016/j.ejso.2006.11.006

Gross, E.R., & Groce, D.F. (1998). An evaluation of nitrile gloves as an alternative to natural rubber latex for handling chemotherapeutic agents. *Journal of Oncology Pharmacy Practice, 4,* 165–168. doi:10.1177/107815529800400305

Gulati, S., Pokhariyal, S., Sharma, R.K., Elhence, R., Kher, V., Pandey, C.M., & Gupta, A. (2001). Pulse cyclophosphamide therapy in frequently relapsing nephritic syndrome. *Nephrology, Dialysis, Transplantation, 16,* 2013–2017. doi:10.1093/ndt/16.10.2013

Guthrie, B., Rouster-Stevens, K.A., & Reynolds, S.L. (2007). Review of medications used in juvenile rheumatoid arthritis. *Pediatric Emergency Care, 23,* 38–46. doi:10.1097/PEC.0b013e31802c61ae

Hales, B.F., Smith, S., & Robaire, B. (1986). Cyclophosphamide in the seminal fluid of treated males: Transmission to females by mating and effect on pregnancy outcome. *Toxicology and Applied Pharmacology, 84,* 423–430.

Hansel, S., Castegnaro, M., Sportouch, M.H., De Meo, M., Milhavet, J.C., Laget, M., & Dumenil, G. (1997). Chemical degradation of wastes of antineoplastic agents: Cyclophosphamide, ifosfamide, and melphalan. *International Archives of Occupational and Environmental Health, 69,* 109–114.

Hansen, J., & Olsen, J.H. (1994). Cancer morbidity among Danish female pharmacy technicians. *Scandinavian Journal of Work and Environmental Health, 20,* 22–26.

Harris, J.P., Weisman, M.H., Derebery, J.M., Espeland, M.A., Gantz, B.J., Gulya, J.A., ... Brookhouser, P.E. (2003). Treatment of corticosteroid-responsive autoimmune inner ear disease with methotrexate: A randomized controlled trial. *JAMA, 290,* 1975–1883. doi:10.1001/jama.290.14.1875

Harris, P.E., Connor, T.H., Stevens, K.R., & Theiss, J.C. (1992). Cytogenetic assessment of occupational exposure of nurses to antineoplastic agents. *Journal of Occupational Medicine and Toxicology, 1,* 243–254.

Harrison, B.R., Godefroid, R.J., & Kavanaugh, E.A. (1996). Quality-assurance testing of staff pharmacists handling cytotoxic agents. *American Journal of Health-System Pharmacy, 53,* 402–407.

Harrison, B.R., & Kloos, M.D. (1999). Penetration and splash protection of six disposable gown materials against fifteen antineoplastic drugs. *Journal of Oncology Pharmacy Practice, 5,* 61–66. doi:10.1177/107815529900500201

Harrison, B.R., Peters, B.G., & Bing, M.R. (2006). Comparison of surface contamination with cyclophosphamide and fluorouracil using a closed-system drug transfer device versus standard preparation techniques. *American Journal of Health-System Pharmacy, 63,* 1736–1744.

Hayden, B.C., Jockovich, M.E., Murray, T.G., Voigt, M., Milne, P., Kralinger, M., ... Parel, J.M. (2004). Pharmacokinetics of systemic versus focal carboplatin chemotherapy in the rabbit eye: Possible implication in the treatment of retinoblastoma. *Investigative Ophthalmology and Visual Science, 45,* 3644–3649. doi:10.1167/iovs.04-0228

Hedmer, M., Jonsson, B.A.G., & Nygren, O. (2004). Development and validation of methods for environmental monitoring of cyclophosphamide in workplaces. *Journal of Environmental Monitoring, 6,* 979–984. doi:10.1039/B409277E

Hemminki, K., Kyyronen, P., & Lindbohm, M.L. (1985). Spontaneous abortions and malformations in the offspring of nurses exposed to anaesthetic gases, cytostatic drugs, and other potential hazards in hospitals, based on registered information of outcome. *Journal of Epidemiology and Community Health, 39,* 141–147.

Hirst, M., Tse, S., Mills, D.G., Levin, L., & White, D.F. (1984). Occupational exposure to cyclophosphamide. *Lancet, 1,* 186–188.

Ho, D. (2008, October 3). Nanodiamond drug delivery system could revolutionize cancer treatment. Retrieved from http://nextbigfuture.com/2008/10/nanodiamond-drug-delivery-system-could.html

Hydrik, C. (2009). Treatment of ovarian cancer with IP chemotherapy. *Oncology: Nurse Edition, 23*(Suppl. 11), 18–20.

Ikeda, K., Yagi, Y., Takegami, M., Lu, Y., Morimoto, K., & Kurokawa, N. (2007). Efforts to ensure safety of hospital pharmacy personnel occupationally exposed to antineoplastic drugs during a preparation task. *Hospital Pharmacy, 42,* 209–218.

International Agency for Research on Cancer. (2006). *IARC monographs on the evaluation of carcinogenic risks to humans.* Retrieved from http://monographs.iarc.fr/ENG/Preamble/CurrentPreamble.pdf

International Organization for Standardization. (1999). *ISO 14644-1: Cleanrooms and associated controlled environments—Part 1: Classification of air cleanliness.* Geneva, Switzerland: Author.

Johnson, E.G., & Janosik, J.E. (1989). Manufacturers' recommendations for handling spilled antineoplastic agents. *American Journal of Hospital Pharmacy, 46,* 318–319.

Kaparissides, C., Alexandridou, S., Kotti, K., & Chaitidou, S. (2006). Recent advances in novel drug delivery systems. *Journal of Nanotechnology Online, 2.* doi:10.2240/azojono0111

Kaufman, M.B. (2009, April). To crush or not to crush: Do your homework before breaking down medications. *The Hospitalist.* Retrieved from http://www.the-hospitalist.org/details/article/184167/To_Crush_or_Not_to_Crush__.html

Kendall, A., Gillmore, R., & Newlands, E. (2003). Chemotherapy for trophoblastic disease: Current standards. *Expert Review of Anticancer Therapy, 3,* 48–54.

Kiffmeyer, T.K., Kube, C., Opiolka, S., Schmidt, K.G., Schoppe, G., & Sessink, P.J.M. (2002). Vapour pressures, evaporation behaviour and airborne concentrations of hazardous drugs: Implications for occupational safety. *Pharmaceutical Journal, 268,* 331–337.

Knowles, M.S., Holton, E.F., III, & Swanson, R.A. (2005). *The adult learner: The definitive classic in adult education and human resource development* (6th ed.). Burlington, MA: Elsevier.

Kolb, D.A. (1984). *Experiential learning: Experience as the source of learning and development.* Englewood Cliffs, NJ: Prentice-Hall.

Krepinsky, A., Bryant, D.W., Davison, L., Young, B., Heddle, J., McCalla, D.R., ... Michalko, K. (1990). Comparison of three assays for genetic effect of antineoplastic drugs on cancer patients and their nurses. *Environmental and Molecular Mutagenesis, 15,* 83–92.

Kromhout, H., Hoek, F., Uitterhoeve, R., Huijbers, R., Overmars, R.F., Anzion, R.B., & Vermeulen, R. (2000). Postulating a dermal pathway for exposure to anti-neoplastic drugs among hospital workers: Applying a conceptual model to the results of three workplace surveys. *Annals of Occupational Hygiene, 44,* 551–560.

Kunwar, S., Prados, M.D., Chang, S.M., Berger, M.S., Lang, F.F., Piepmeier, J.M., ... Puri, R.K. (2007). Direct intracerebral delivery of cintredekin besudotox (IL13-PE38QQR) in recurrent malignant glioma: A report by the Cintredekin Besudotox Intraparenchymal Study Group. *Journal of Clinical Oncology, 25,* 837–844. doi:10.1200/JCO.2006.08.1117

Labuhn, K., Valanis, B., Schoeny, R., Loveday, K., & Vollmer, W.M. (1998). Nurses' and pharmacists' exposure to antineoplastic drugs: Findings from industrial hygiene scans and urine mutagenicity tests. *Cancer Nursing, 21,* 79–89.

Ladik, C., Stoehr, G., & Maurer, M. (1980). Precautionary measures in the preparation of antineoplastics. *American Journal of Hospital Pharmacy, 37,* 1184–1186.

Larson, D.A., Rubenstein, J.L., & McDermott, M.W. (2008). Metastatic cancer to the brain. In V.T. DeVita Jr., T.S. Lawrence, & S.A. Rosenberg (Eds.), *Cancer: Principles and practice of oncology* (8th ed., Vol. 2, pp. 2461–2475). Philadelphia, PA: Lippincott Williams & Wilkins.

Larson, R.R., Khazaeli, M.B., & Dillon, H.K. (2003a). Development of an HPLC method for simultaneous analysis of five antineoplastic agents. *Applied Occupational and Environmental Hygiene, 18,* 109–119.

Larson, R.R., Khazaeli, M.B., & Dillon, H.K. (2003b). A new monitoring method using solid sorbent media for evaluation of airborne cyclophosphamide and other antineoplastic agents. *Applied Occupational and Environmental Hygiene, 18,* 120–131.

Lasak, J.M., Sataloff, R.T., Hawkshaw, M., Carey, T.E., Lyons, K.M., & Spiegel, J.R. (2001). Autoimmune inner ear disease: Steroid and cytotoxic drug therapy. *Ear, Nose, and Throat Journal, 80,* 808–811, 815–816, 818. Retrieved from http://www.thefreelibrary.com/_/print/PrintArticle .aspx?id=80845987

Lauwerys, R. (1984). Objectives of biological monitoring in occupational health practice. In A. Aitio, V. Riihimaki, & H. Vainio (Eds.), *Biologic monitoring and surveillance of workers exposed to chemicals* (pp. 3–6). Washington, DC: Hemisphere.

Libutti, S.K., Saltz, L.B., & Tepper, J.E. (2008). Cancers of the gastrointestinal tract: Colon cancer. In V.T. DeVita Jr., T.S. Lawrence, & S.A. Rosenberg (Eds.), *Cancer: Principles and practice of oncology* (8th ed., Vol. 1, pp. 1232–1284). Philadelphia, PA: Lippincott Williams & Wilkins.

Mader, R.R.M., Rizovski, B.B., Steger, G.G.G., Wachter, A.A., Kotz, R.R., & Rainer, H.H. (1996). Exposure of oncologic nurses to methotrexate in the treatment of osteosarcoma. *Archives of Environmental Health, 51,* 310–314.

Mahon, S.M, Casperson, D.S., Yackzan, S., Goodner, S., Hasse, B., Hawkins, J., ... Witcher, V. (1994). Safe handling practices of cytotoxic drugs: The results of a chapter survey. *Oncology Nursing Forum, 21,* 1157–1165.

Mallick, I. (2007). Cutaneous T-cell lymphoma—Treatment options. Retrieved from http://lymphoma.about.com/od/treatment/p/ctcltreatment.htm

Maluf, S.W., & Erdtmann, B. (2000). Follow-up study of the genetic damage in lymphocytes of pharmacists and nurses handling antineoplastic drugs evaluated by cytokinesis-block micronuclei analysis and single cell gel electrophoresis assay. *Mutation Research, 471,* 21–27. doi:10.1016/S1383-5718(00)00107-8

Mardor, Y., Rahav, O., Zauberman, Y., Lidar, Z., Ocherashvilli, A., Daniels, D., ... Ram, Z. (2005). Convection-enhanced drug delivery: Increased efficacy and magnetic resonance image monitoring. *Cancer Research, 65,* 6858–6863. doi:10.1158/0008-5472.CAN-05-0161

Margolin, J.F., & Poplack, D.G. (2008). Leukemias and lymphomas of childhood. In V.T. DeVita Jr., T.S. Lawrence, & S.A. Rosenberg (Eds.), *Cancer: Principles and practice of oncology* (8th ed., Vol. 2, pp. 2085–2097). Philadelphia, PA: Lippincott Williams & Wilkins.

Martin, S. (2005a). The adverse health effects of occupational exposure to hazardous drugs. *Community Oncology, 2,* 397–400.

Martin, S. (2005b). Chemotherapy handling and effects among nurses and their offspring [Abstract]. *Oncology Nursing Forum, 32,* 425.

Martin, S. (2006). Outpatient nurses' perception of chemotherapy handling risks. *Oncology Nursing Forum, 33,* Abstract No. 252. Retrieved from http://onsopcontent.ons.org/meetings/2006abstracts/CongressAbs/abstract252.shtml

Martin, S., & Larson, E. (2003). Chemotherapy-handling practices of outpatient and office-based oncology nurses. *Oncology Nursing Forum, 30,* 575–581. doi:10.1188/03.ONF.575-581

Mason, H.J., Blair, S., Sams, C., Jones, K., Garfitt, S.J., Cuschieri, M.J., & Baxter, P.J. (2005). Exposure to antineoplastic drugs in two UK hospital pharmacy units. *Annals of Occupational Hygiene, 49,* 603–610. doi:10.1093/annhyg/mei023

Matthews, E., Snell, K., & Coats, H. (2006). Intra-arterial chemotherapy for limb preservation in patients with osteosarcoma: Nursing implications. *Clinical Journal of Oncology Nursing, 10,* 581–589. doi:10.1188/06.CJON.581-589

McDevitt, J.J., Lees, P.S.J., & McDiarmid, M.A. (1993). Exposure of hospital pharmacists and nurses to antineoplastic agents. *Journal of Occupational Medicine, 35,* 57–60.

McDiarmid, M., & Emmett, E. (1987). Biological monitoring and medical surveillance of workers exposed to antineoplastic agents. *Seminars in Occupational Medicine, 2,* 109–117.

McDiarmid, M.A. (1990). Medical surveillance for antineoplastic drug handlers. *American Journal of Hospital Pharmacy, 47,* 1061–1066.

McDiarmid, M.A., & Condon, M. (2005). Organizational safety culture/climate and worker compliance with hazardous drug guidelines: Lessons from the blood-borne pathogen experience. *Journal of Occupational and Environmental Medicine, 47,* 740–749.

McDiarmid, M.A., & Curbow, B. (1992). Risk communication and surveillance approaches for workplace reproductive hazards. *Journal of Occupational Medicine and Toxicology, 1,* 63–74.

McDiarmid, M.A., Oliver, M.S., Roth, T.S., Rogers, B., & Escalante, C. (2010). Chromosome 5 and 7 abnormalities in oncology personnel handling anticancer drugs. *Journal of Occupational and Environmental Medicine, 52,* 1028–1034.

McDonald, C.E. (2007). Intraoperative intravesical epirubicin: Implementing the process. *Urologic Nursing, 27,* 210–212.

Mehta, M.P., Buckner, J., Sawaya, R.P., & Cannon, G.M. (2008). Neoplasms of the central nervous system. In V.T. DeVita Jr., T.S. Lawrence, & S.A. Rosenberg (Eds.), *Cancer: Principles and practice of oncology* (8th ed., Vol. 2, pp. 1975–2032). Philadelphia, PA: Lippincott Williams & Wilkins.

Meijster, T., Fransman, W., Veldhof, R., & Kromhout, H. (2006). Exposure to antineoplastic drugs outside the hospital environment. *Annals of Occupational Hygiene, 50,* 657–664. doi:10.1093/annhyg/mel023

Minoia, C., Turci, R., Sottani, C., Schiavi, A., Perbellini, L., Angeleri, S., … Apostoli, P. (1998). Application of high performance liquid chromatography/tandem mass spectrometry in the environmental and biological monitoring of health care personnel occupationally exposed to cyclophosphamide and ifosfamide. *Rapid Communications in Mass Spectrometry, 12,* 1485–1493. doi:10.1002/(SICI)1097-0231(19981030)12:20<1485::AID-RCM333>3.0.CO;2-N

Mitchell, J.F. (2010, July). Oral dosage forms that should not be crushed. Retrieved from http://www.ismp.org/Tools/DoNotCrush.pdf

Muehlbauer, P.M., Klapec, K., Locklin, J., George, M.E., Cunningham, L., Gottschalk, C., & Seidel, G.D. (2006). Part II: Nursing implications of administering chemotherapy in interventional radiology or the operating room. *Clinical Journal of Oncology Nursing, 10,* 345–356. doi:10.1188/06.CJON.345-356

Mulvihill, A., Budning, A., Jay, V., Vandenhoven, C., Heon, E., Gallie, B.L., & Chan, H.S. (2003). Ocular motility changes after subtenon carboplatin chemotherapy for retinoblastoma. *Archives of Ophthalmology, 121,* 1120–1124. doi:10.1001/archopht.121.8.1120

Muthu, M.S., & Singh, S. (2009). Targeted nanomedicines: Effective treatment modalities for cancer, AIDS and brain disorders. *Nanomedicine, 4,* 105–118. doi:10.2217/17435889.4.1.105

National Cancer Institute. (1998). Cutaneous T-cell lymphoma (PDQ®). Retrieved from http://www.meds.com/pdq/tcell_pro.html

National Cancer Institute. (2006, January 5). NCI clinical announcement: Intraperitoneal chemotherapy for ovarian cancer. Retrieved from http://ctep.cancer.gov/highlights/docs/clin_annc_010506.pdf

National Cancer Institute. (2008, January). Skin cancer treatment (PDQ®) [Health professional version]. Retrieved from http://www.cancer.gov/cancertopics/pdq/treatment/skin/HealthProfessional

National Institute for Occupational Safety and Health. (1996). Summary for respirator users. Retrieved from http://www.cdc.gov/niosh/respsumm.html

National Institute for Occupational Safety and Health. (2004, September). *NIOSH alert: Preventing occupational exposure to antineoplastic and other hazardous drugs in health care settings* (NIOSH Publication No. 2004-165). Retrieved from http://www.cdc.gov/niosh/docs/2004-165

National Institute for Occupational Safety and Health. (2007). *Workplace solution: Medical surveillance for health care workers exposed to hazardous drugs* (NIOSH Publication No. 2007-117). Retrieved from http://www.cdc.gov/niosh/docs/wp-solutions/2007-117

National Institutes of Health. (1994). Recommendations for the safe handling of cytotoxic drugs. Retrieved from http://www.cc.nih.gov/nursing/shhdpro.html

Nehring, W.M., & Lashley, F.R. (Eds.). (2010). *High-fidelity patient simulation in nursing education.* Sudbury, MA: Jones and Bartlett.

Nieweg, R.M., de Boer, M., Dubbleman, R.C., Gall, H.E., Hesselman, G.M., Lenssen, P.C., … Slegt, J.H. (1994). Safe handling of antineoplastic drugs. Results of a survey. *Cancer Nursing, 17,* 501–511.

Niland, J. (1994). Industrial hygiene. In C. Zenz (Ed.), *Occupational medicine* (3rd ed., pp. 1045–1050). St. Louis, MO: Mosby.

Notarianni, M.A., Curry-Lourenco, K., Barham, P., & Palmer, K. (2009). Engaging learners across generations: The Progressive Professional Development Model. *Journal of Continuing Education in Nursing, 40,* 261–266.

Novartis Pharmaceuticals Corp. (2009). *Gleevec®* [Package insert]. Retrieved from http://www.pharma.us.novartis.com/product/pi/pdf/gleevec_tabs.pdf

NSF International/American National Standards Institute. (2009, April 20). *NSF 49 class II (laminar flow) biosafety cabinetry* (10th ed.). Ann Arbor, MI: NSF International.

NuAire, Inc. (2005). Containment capabilities of a class II, type A2 BSC using a chemo pad on the worksurface. Retrieved from http://www.nuaire.com/download/whitepaper/containment _capabilities.pdf

Nygren, O., & Aspman, O. (2004). Validation and application of wipe sampling and portable XRF analysis as an on-site screening method for assessment of deposited aerosols in workplaces . *Australian Journal of Chemistry, 57,* 1021–1028. doi:10.1071/CH04126

Nygren, O., Gustavsson, B., & Eriksson, R. (2005). A test method for assessment of spill and leakage from drug preparation systems. *Annals of Occupational Hygiene, 49,* 711–718.

Nygren, O., Gustavsson, B., Strom, L., & Friberg, A. (2002). Cisplatin contamination observed on the outside of drug vials. *Annals of Occupational Hygiene, 46,* 555–557.

Nygren, O., & Lundgren, C. (1997). Determination of platinum in workroom air and in blood and urine from nursing staff attending patients receiving cisplatin chemotherapy. *International Archives of Occupational and Environmental Health, 70,* 209–214. doi:10.1007/s004200050209

Nygren, O., Olofsson, E., & Johannson, L. (2008). Spill and leakage using a drug preparation system based on double-filter technology. *Annals of Occupational Hygiene, 52,* 95–98.

Nygren, O., Olofsson, E., & Johannson, L. (2009). NIOSH definition of closed-system drug-transfer devices. *Annals of Occupational Hygiene, 53,* 549.

Occupational Safety and Health Administration. (1992/2008). Bloodborne pathogens standard. 29 CFR 1910.1030. Retrieved from http://www.osha.gov/pls/oshaweb/owadisp. show_document?p_table=STANDARDS&p_id=10051

Occupational Safety and Health Administration. (1995, September 22). Section VI, Chapter 2: Controlling occupational exposure to hazardous drugs. In *OSHA technical manual.* Retrieved from http://www.osha.gov/dts/osta/otm/otm_vi/otm_vi_2.html

Occupational Safety and Health Administration. (1998). Informational booklet on industrial hygiene. Retrieved from http://www.osha.gov/Publications/OSHA3143/OSHA3143.htm#Industrial

Occupational Safety and Health Administration. (2002). Guidelines for laundry in health care facilities. Retrieved from http://www.cdc.gov/od/ohs/biosfty/laundry.htm

Oesch, F., Hengstler, J.G., Arand, M., & Fuchs, J. (1995). Detection of primary DNA damage: Applicability to biomonitoring of genotoxic occupational exposure and in clinical therapy. *Pharmacogenetics, 5*(Special Issue), S118–S122.

Oestreicher, U., Stephan, G., & Glatzel, M. (1990). Chromosome and SCE analysis in peripheral lymphocytes of persons occupationally exposed to cytostatic drugs handled with and without use of safety covers. *Mutation Research, 242,* 271–277.

Parra, S.A. (2000). Cytotoxic chemotherapy in the treatment of nonmalignant disease. *Journal of Intravenous Nursing, 23,* 359–365.

Patel, T.B. (2007). Recent trends in brain targeted drug delivery systems: An overview. *Pharmaceutical Reviews, 5*(2). Retrieved from http://www.pharmainfo.net/reviews/recent-trends-brain-targeted-drug-delivery-systemsan-overview

Pestieau, S.R., Schnake, K.J., Stuart, O.A., & Sugarbaker, P.H. (2001). Impact of carrier solutions on pharmacokinetics of intraperitoneal chemotherapy. *Cancer Chemotherapy and Pharmacology, 47,* 269–276. doi:10.1007/s002800000214

Peters, G.F., McKeon, M.R., & Weiss, W.T. (2007). Potential for airborne contamination in turbulent- and unidirectional-airflow compounding aseptic isolators. *American Journal of Health-System Pharmacy, 64,* 622–631. doi:10.2146/ajhp060067

Pethran, A., Schierl, R., Hauff, K., Grimm, C.-H., Boos, K.-S., & Nowak, D. (2003). Uptake of antineoplastic agents in pharmacy and hospital personnel. Part I: Monitoring of urinary concentrations. *International Archives of Occupational and Environmental Health, 76,* 5–10. doi:10.1007/s00420-002-0383-8

Petralia, S.A., Dosemeci, M., Adams, E.E., & Zahm, S.H. (1999). Cancer mortality among women employed in health care occupations in 24 U.S. states, 1984–1993. *American Journal of Industrial Medicine, 36,* 159–165. doi:10.1002/(SICI)1097-0274(199907)36:1<159::AID-AJIM23>3.0.CO;2-K

Pfizer Inc. (2010). *Sutent®* [Package insert]. Retrieved from http://www.pfizer.com/files/products/uspi_sutent.pdf

Pingpank, J.F., Jr. (2008). Diagnosis and treatment of peritoneal carcinomatosis. In V.T. DeVita Jr., T.S. Lawrence, & S.A. Rosenberg (Eds.), *Cancer: Principles and practice of oncology* (8th ed., Vol. 2, pp. 2389–2400). Philadelphia, PA: Lippincott Williams & Wilkins.

Polovich, M. (2004). Safe handling of hazardous drugs. *Online Journal of Issues in Nursing, 9*(3). Retrieved from http://nursingworld.org/MainMenuCategories/ANAMarketplace/ANAPeriodicals/OJIN/TableofContents/Volume92004/No3Sept04/HazardousDrugs.aspx

Polovich, M. (2010). *Nurses' use of hazardous drug safe handling precautions.* Unpublished doctoral dissertation, Georgia State University, Atlanta.

Polovich, M., Whitford, J.M., & Olsen, M. (Eds.). (2009). *Chemotherapy and biotherapy guidelines and recommendations for practice* (3rd ed.). Pittsburgh, PA: Oncology Nursing Society.

Raghavan, D. (2009). Neoadjuvant chemotherapy for urothelial bladder cancer. Retrieved from http://www.uptodate.com

Rekhadevi, P.V., Sailaja, N., Chandrasekhar, M., Mahboob, M., Rahman, M.F., & Grover, P. (2007). Genotoxicity assessment in oncology nurses handling anti-neoplastic drugs. *Mutagenesis, 22,* 395–401. doi:10.1093/mutage/gem032

Roberts, S., Khammo, N., McDonnell, G., & Sewell, G.J. (2006). Studies on the decontamination of surfaces exposed to cytotoxic drugs in chemotherapy workstations. *Journal of Oncology Pharmacy Practice, 12,* 95–104. doi:10.1177/1078155206070439

Rogers, B., & Emmett, E.A. (1987). Handling antineoplastic agents: Urine mutagenicity in nurses. *Image: The Journal of Nursing Scholarship, 19,* 108–113.

Roth, A.D., Berney, C.R., Rohner, S., Allal, A.S., Morel, P., Marti, M.C., … Alberto, P. (2000). Intra-arterial chemotherapy for locally advanced or recurrent carcinomas of the penis and anal canal: An active treatment modality with curative potential. *British Journal of Cancer, 83,* 1637–1642. doi:10.1054/bjoc.2000.1525

Rubino, F.M., Floridia, L., Pietropaolo, A.M., Tavazzani, M., & Colombi, A. (1999). Measurement of surface contamination by certain antineoplastic drugs using high-performance liquid chromatography: Applications in occupational hygiene investigations in hospital environments. *La Medicina del Lavoro, 90,* 572–583.

Rundback, J.H., Gray, R.J., Buck, D.R., Dolmatch, B.L., Haffner, G.H., Horton, K.M., … Sugarbaker, P.H. (1994). Fluoroscopically guided peritoneal catheter placement for intraperitoneal chemotherapy. *Journal of Vascular and Interventional Radiology, 5,* 161–165.

Sampson, J.H., Akabani, G., Friedman, A.H., Bigner, D., Kunwar, S., Berger, M.S., & Bankiewicz, K.S. (2006). Comparison of intratumoral bolus injection and convection-enhanced delivery of radiolabeled antitenascin monoclonal antibodies. *Neurosurgical Focus, 20*(4), E14. doi:10.3171/foc.2006.20.4.9

Saurel-Cubizolles, M.J., Job-Spira, N., & Estryn-Behar, M. (1993). Ectopic pregnancy and occupational exposure to antineoplastic drugs. *Lancet, 341,* 1169–1171. doi:10.1016/0140-6736(93)91000-C

Schmaus, G., Schierl, R., & Funck, S. (2002). Monitoring surface contamination by antineoplastic drugs using gas chromatography-mass spectrometry and voltammetry. *American Journal of Health-System Pharmacy, 59,* 956–961.

Selevan, S.G., Lindbohm, M.L., Hornung, R.W., & Hemminki, K. (1985). A study of occupational exposure to antineoplastic drugs and fetal loss in nurses. *New England Journal of Medicine, 313,* 1173–1178.

Sessink, P.J., Boer, K.A., Scheefhals, A.P., Anzion, R.B., & Bos, R.P. (1992). Occupational exposure to antineoplastic agents at several departments in a hospital. Environmental contamination and excretion of cyclophosphamide and ifosfamide in urine of exposed workers. *International Archives of Occupational and Environmental Health, 64,* 105–112.

Sessink, P.J., Kroese, E.D., van Kranen, H.J., & Bos, R.P. (1995). Cancer risk assessment for health care workers occupationally exposed to cyclophosphamide. *International Archives of Occupational and Environmental Health, 67,* 317–323.

Sessink, P.J., Van de Kerkhof, M.C.A., Anzion, R.B., Noordhoek, J., & Bos, R.P. (1994). Environmental contamination and assessment of exposure to antineoplastic agents by determination of cyclophosphamide in urine of exposed pharmacy technicians: Is skin absorption an important exposure route? *Archives of Environmental Health, 49,* 165–169.

Sessink, P.J., Wittenhorst, B.C.J., Anzion, R.B., & Bos, R.P. (1997). Exposure of pharmacy technicians to antineoplastic agents: Reevaluation after additional protective measures. *Archives of Environmental Health, 52,* 240–244.

Sessink, P.J.M., Rolf, M.E., & Ryden, N.S. (1999). Evaluation of the PhaSeal hazardous drug containment system. *Hospital Pharmacy, 34,* 1311–1317.

Shipp, M.A., & Harris, N.L. (2000). Non-Hodgkin's lymphomas. In L. Goldman & J.C. Bennett (Eds.), *Cecil textbook of medicine* (21st ed., pp. 962–969). Philadelphia, PA: Saunders.

Shoji, T., Tanaka, F., Yanagihara, K., Inui, K., & Wada, H. (2002). Phase II study of repeated intrapleural chemotherapy using implantable access system for management of malignant pleural effusion. *Chest, 121,* 821–824. doi:10.1378/chest.121.3.821

Shortridge, L.A., Lemasters, G.K., Valanis, B., & Hertzberg, V. (1995). Menstrual cycles in nurses handling antineoplastic drugs. *Cancer Nursing, 18,* 439–444.

Singleton, L.C., & Connor, T.H. (1999). An evaluation of the permeability of chemotherapy gloves to three cancer chemotherapy drugs. *Oncology Nursing Forum, 26,* 1491–1496.

Skov, T., Lynge, E., Maarup, B., Olsen, J., Rørth, M., & Winthereik, H. (1990). Risks for physicians handling antineoplastic drugs. *Lancet, 336,* 1446.

Skov, T., Maarup, B., Olsen, J., Rorth, M., Winthereik, H., & Lynge, E. (1992). Leukaemia and reproductive outcome among nurses handling antineoplastic drugs. *British Journal of Industrial Medicine, 49,* 855–861.

Smolen, J.S., Aletaha, D., Koeller, M., Weisman, M.H., & Emery, P. (2007). New therapies for treament of rheumatoid arthritis. *Lancet, 370,* 1861–1874. doi:10.1016/S0140-6736(07)60784-3

Sotaniemi, E.A., Sutinen, S., Arranto, A.J., Sutinen, S., Sotaniemi, K.A., Lehtola, J., & Pelkonen, R.O. (1983). Liver damage in nurses handling cytostatic agents. *Acta Medica Scandinavica, 214,* 181–189.

Srinivasan, S., & Slomovic, A.R. (2007). Sjögren syndrome. *Comprehensive Ophthalmology Update, 8,* 205–212.

Stern, S.T., & McNeil, S.E. (2008). Nanotechnology safety concerns revisited. *Toxicological Sciences, 101,* 4–21. doi:10.1093/toxsci/kfm169

Stücker, I., Caillard, J.F., Collin, R., Gout, M., Poyen, D., & Hemon, D. (1990). Risk of spontaneous abortion among nurses handling antineoplastic drugs. *Scandinavian Journal of Work, Environment and Health, 16,* 102–107.

Stücker, I., Mandereau, L., & Hémon, D. (1993). Relationship between birthweight and occupational exposure to cytostatic drugs during or before pregnancy. *Scandinavian Journal of Work, Environment and Health, 19,* 148–153.

Sugarbaker, P.H. (1998). *Management of peritoneal surface malignancy using intraperitoneal chemotherapy and cytoreductive surgery: A manual for physicians and nurses* (3rd ed.). Grand Rapids, MI: Ludann. Retrieved from http://www.surgicaloncology.com/gpmtitle.htm

Sugarbaker, P.H., Klecker, R.W., Gianola, F.J., & Speyer, J.L. (1986). Prolonged treatment schedules with intraperitoneal 5-fluorouracil diminish the local-regional nature of drug distribution. *American Journal of Clinical Oncology, 9,* 1–7.

Sugarbaker, P.H., & Stephens, A.D. (n.d.). Pharacokinetics of intraperitoneal chemotherapy. In *Atlas of appendix cancer and pseudomyxoma peritonei.* Retrieved from http://www.surgicaloncology.com/atpharms.htm

Sutton, A. (2004, September). Needleless chemotherapy: Safety and efficacy of aerosolized chemotherapy being studied in young patients with cancer. *OncoLog, 69*(9). Retrieved from http://www2.mdanderson.org/depts/oncolog

Tatsumura, T., Koyama, S., Tsujimoto, M., Kitagawa, M., & Kagamimori, S. (1993). Further study of nebulisation chemotherapy, a new chemotherapeutic method in the treatment of lung carcinomas: Fundamental and clinical. *British Journal of Cancer, 68,* 1146–1149.

Testa, A., Gianchella, M., Palma, S., Appolloni, M., Padua, L., Tranfo, G., ... Cozzi, R. (2007). Occupational exposure to antineoplastic agents induces a high level of chromosome damage. Lack of an effect of GST polymorphisms. *Toxicology and Applied Pharmacology, 223,* 46–55. doi:10.1016/j.taap.2007.05.006

Thiringer, G., Granung, G., Holmén, A., Högstedt, B., Järvholm, B., Jönsson, D., ... Westin, J. (1991). Comparison of methods for the biomonitoring of nurses handling antitumor drugs. *Scandinavian Journal of Work, Environment and Health, 17,* 133–138.

Thomson Reuters Micromedex® 2.0. (2009). Retrieved from http://www.thomsonhc.com

Turkoski, B.B., Lance, B.R., & Tomsik, E.A. (Eds.). (2009). *Drug information handbook for nursing* (11th ed.). Hudson, OH: LexiComp.

Undeger, U., Basaran, N., Kars, A., & Guc, D. (1999). Assessment of DNA damage in handling antineoplastic drugs by the alkaline COMET assay. *Mutation Research, 439,* 277–285.

U.S. Bureau of Labor Statistics. (2009). May 2009 national occupational employment and wage estimates, United States. Retrieved from http://www.bls.gov/oes/current/oes_nat.htm

U.S. Department of Health and Human Services, Public Health Service, National Toxicology Program. (2010). *Report on carcinogens.* Retrieved from http://ntp.niehs.nih.gov/go/roc

U.S. Environmental Protection Agency. (2008, April 14). Epinephrine syringe and epinephrine salts. Retrieved from http://yosemite.epa.gov/osw/rcra.nsf/0c994248c239947e85256d090071175f/6a5dedf2fba24fe68525744b0045b4af!OpenDocument

U.S. Environmental Protection Agency. (2009). Solid waste disposal. 42 U.S.C. 6903(5).

U.S. Environmental Protection Agency. (2010a, January). Medical waste. Retrieved from http://www.epa.gov/waste/nonhaz/industrial/medical/index.htm

U.S. Environmental Protection Agency. (2010b). Residues of hazardous waste in empty containers. 40 CFR 261.7. Retrieved from http://ecfr.gpoaccess.gov/cgi/t/text/text-idx?c=ecfr&sid=4d05bc1997664246015a8364e117bbd2&rgn=div8&view=text&node=40:25.0.1.1.2.1.1.7&idno=40

U.S. Pharmacopeia. (2008a). Chapter 797: Pharmaceutical compounding—sterile preparations. In *The United States Pharmacopeia,* 31st rev., and The National Formulary, 26th ed. Rockville, MD: Author.

U.S. Pharmacopeia. (2008b). Chapter 1072: Disinfectants and antiseptics. In *The United States Pharmacopeia,* 31st rev, and The National Formulary, 26th ed. Rockville, MD: Author.

U.S. Pharmacopeia. (n.d.). About USP. Retrieved from http://www.usp.org/aboutUSP

Valanis, B., McNeil, V., & Driscoll, K. (1991). Staff members' compliance with their facility's antineoplastic drug handling policy. *Oncology Nursing Form, 18,* 571–576.

Valanis, B., Vollmer, W., Labuhn, K., & Glass, A. (1997). Occupational exposure to antineoplastic agents and self-reported infertility among nurses and pharmacists. *Journal of Occupational and Environmental Medicine, 39,* 574–580.

Valanis, B., Vollmer, W.M., Labuhn, K., Glass, A., & Corelle, C. (1992). Antineoplastic drug handling protection after OSHA guidelines. Comparison by profession, handling activity, and work site. *Journal of Occupational Medicine, 34,* 149–155.

Valanis, B., Vollmer, W.M., & Steele, P. (1999). Occupational exposure to antineoplastic agents: Self-reported miscarriages and stillbirths among nurses and pharmacists. *Journal of Occupational and Environmental Medicine, 41,* 632–638.

Valanis, B.G., Vollmer, W.M., Labuhn, K.T., & Glass, A.G. (1993a). Acute symptoms associated with antineoplastic drug handling among nurses. *Cancer Nursing, 16,* 288–295.

Valanis, B.G., Vollmer, W.M., Labuhn, K.T., & Glass, A.G. (1993b). Association of antineoplastic drug handling with acute adverse effects in pharmacy personnel. *American Journal of Hospital Pharmacy, 50,* 455–462.

Van der Speeten, K., Stuart, O.A., Mahteme, H., & Sugarbaker, P.H. (2009). A pharmacologic analysis of intraoperative intracavitary cancer chemotherapy with doxorubicin. *Cancer Chemotherapy and Pharmacology, 63,* 799–805. doi:10.1007/s00280-008-0800-0

Vandenbroucke, J. (2001). Quality assurance project in a university hospital—2 years of experience. *European Journal of Hospital Pharmacy Practice, 7*(2), 60–68.

Verity, R., Wiseman, T., Ream, E., Teasdale, E., & Richardson, A. (2008). Exploring the work of nurses who administer chemotherapy. *European Journal of Oncology Nursing, 12,* 244–252. doi:10.1016/j.ejon.2008.02.001.

Visco, A.G., Meyer, L., Xi, S., & Brown, C.G. (2009). One disease, two lives: Exploring the treatment of breast cancer during pregnancy. *Clinical Journal of Oncology Nursing, 13,* 426–432. doi:10.1188/09.CJON.426-432

Walker, S.J., & Bryden, G. (2010). Managing pleural effusions. *Clinical Journal of Oncology Nursing, 14,* 59–64. doi:10.1188/10.CJON.59-64

Wallemacq, P.E., Capron, A., Vanbinst, R., Boeckmans, E., Gillard, J., & Favier, B. (2006). Permeability of 13 different gloves to 13 cytotoxic agents under controlled dynamic conditions. *American Journal of Health-System Pharmacy, 63,* 547–556. doi:10.2146/ajhp050197

Walusiak, J., Wittczak, T., Ruta, U., & Palczynski. (2002). Occupational asthma due to mitoxantrone. *Allergy, 57,* 461. doi:10.1034/j.1398-9995.2002.13455.x

Washburn, D.J. (2007). Intravesical antineoplastic therapy following transurethral resection of bladder tumors: Nursing implications from the operating room to discharge. *Clinical Journal of Oncology Nursing, 11,* 553–559. doi:10.1188/07.CJON.553-559

Weingart, S.N., Brown, E., Bach, P.B., Eng, K., Johnson, S.A., Kuzel, T.M., ... Walters, R.S. (2008). NCCN Task Force Report: Oral chemotherapy. *Journal of the National Comprehensive Cancer Network, 6*(Suppl. 3), S1–S14.

Welch, J., & Silveira, J.M. (1997). *Safe handling of cytotoxic drugs: An independent study module* (2nd ed.). Pittsburgh, PA: Oncology Nursing Society.

Wesdock, J.C., & Sokas, R.K. (2000). Medical surveillance in work-site safety and health programs. *American Family Physician, 61,* 2785–2790.

Williams, N.T. (2008). Medication administration through enteral feeding tubes. *American Journal of Health-System Pharmacy, 65,* 2347–2357. doi:10.2146/ajhp080155

Wilson, J.P., & Solimando, D.A., Jr. (1981). Aseptic technique as a safety precaution in the preparation of antineoplastic agents. *Hospital Pharmacy, 16,* 575–576, 579–581.

Wittgen, B.P., Kunst, P.W., van der Born, K., van Wijk, A.W., Perkins, W., Pilkiewicz, F.G., ... Postmus, P.E. (2007). Phase I study of aerosolized SLIT cisplatin in the treatment of patients with carcinoma of the lung. *Clinical Cancer Research, 13,* 2414–2421. doi:10.1158/1078-0432.CCR-06-1480

Yan, T.D., Stuart, O.A., Yoo, D., & Sugarbaker, P.H. (2006). Perioperative intraperitoneal chemotherapy for peritoneal surface malignancy. *Journal of Translational Medicine, 4,* Article 17. doi:10.1186/1479-5876-4-17

Yoshida, J., Kosaka, H., Tomioka, K., & Kumagai, S. (2006). Genotoxic risks to nurses from contamination of the work environment with antineoplastic drugs in Japan. *Journal of Occupational Health, 48,* 517–522. doi:10.1539/joh.48.517

Yulan, M., Chunsheng, T., Zeqing, W., Ming, L., Fubo, Y., & Cuiling, S. (2003). Pharmacokinetics of intraperitoneal chemotherapy with continuous washing methods for patients with ovarian cancer. *Progress in Obstetrics and Gynecology, 12,* 158–160. Retrieved from http://journal.shouxi.net/upload/pdf/140/2904/149602_9321.pdf

Zeedijk, M., Greijdanus, B., Steenstra, F.B., & Uges, D.R.A. (2005). Monitoring exposure of cytostatics on the hospital ward: Measuring surface contamination of four different cytostatic drugs from one wipe sample. *European Journal of Hospital Pharmacy Science, 11,* 18–22.

Ziegler, E., Mason, H.J., & Baxter, P.J. (2002). Occupational exposure to cytotoxic drugs in two UK oncology wards. *Occupational and Environmental Medicine, 59,* 608–612. doi:10.1136/oem.59.9.608

SAFE HANDLING OF HAZARDOUS DRUGS, SECOND EDITION   PAGE 83

Appendix A. Hazardous Drug Administration Safe Handling Checklist

Name: _____ Date of Review and Exam: _____

PRIOR TO ADMINISTRATION	Yes	No	Initials
1. Gather equipment required for drug administration.			
2. Select appropriate gloves for hazardous drug administration.			
3. Select appropriate gown for hazardous drug administration.			
4. Identify situations when face shield/eye protection is required.			
5. Locate spill kit and mask.			
6. Obtain hazardous waste container.			
7. Receive drug(s) from pharmacy in sealed container.			
ADMINISTRATION			
1. Wash hands and don gown and gloves before opening drug delivery bag.			
2. Visually inspect the contents of the delivery bag.			
3. Don face shield, as indicated.			
4. Select IV equipment with locking connections.			
5. For IV infusions • Place plastic-backed absorbent pad to protect patient from droplets. • Remove cap from IV tubing and connect to patient delivery site. • Tighten locking connections. • When complete, discontinue IV bag/bottle/tubing intact and recap patient delivery site.			
6. For IV push medications • Wrap gauze around connection to catch drug droplets. • Tighten locking connection. • When complete, remove syringe from needleless connection. • Discard syringe and waste in a puncture-proof/leakproof container.			
7. For intramuscular/subcutaneous injections • Attach needle to syringe. • Tighten locking connection. • When complete, do not recap needle. • Discard syringe-needle unit in puncture-proof/leakproof container.			
8. For oral drugs • Don gloves. • Open unit dose package and place into medicine cup (avoid touching drug or inside of package).			
POST-ADMINISTRATION			
1. Don gown, gloves, and face shield, if indicated.			
2. Seal contact material in plastic bag for transport to hazardous waste container.			
3. Place sealed plastic bag in hazardous waste container.			
4. Remove personal protective equipment properly, seal it in a plastic bag, and dispose of it in the hazardous waste container.			
5. Close lid on waste container.			
6. Wash hands thoroughly after removal and disposal of personal protective equipment.			
7. Decontaminate equipment appropriately in the area.			

Appendix B. Hazardous Drug Administration Practicum for RNs

Objectives	Content	Teaching/Learning Strategies

Recall the properties and health risks of workplace exposure to hazardous drugs.	Characteristics of hazardous drugs
	• Carcinogenicity
	• Reproductive toxicity
	• Teratogenicity or developmental toxicity
	• Infertility
	• Organ toxicity at low doses
	• Genotoxicity
	Drugs similar in structure or toxicity
		• Discussion of clinical scenarios regarding potential exposure
		  – Case study: Nurse attempting to conceive
		  – Case study: Experienced nurse who chooses not to wear personal protective equipment (PPE)
		  – Case study: Explaining to patient and family why you are wearing PPE
		
		Learner will interview nursing staff on their PPE practices in light of current evidence and will evaluate feedback in light of recommended practices.
		
		In advance of clinical experience, learner will download and review National Institute for Occupational Safety and Health's (NIOSH's) 2004 alert, *Preventing Occupational Exposure to Antineoplastic and Other Hazardous Drugs in Health Care Settings* (www.cdc.gov/niosh/docs/2004-165/pdfs/2004-165.pdf).
		
		Materials:
		• NIOSH alert
		• Case studies

Outline potential routes of exposure in the clinical setting.	Potential routes of exposure include • Skin or mucous membrane exposure • Needlesticks or sharps • Inhalation of aerosols, dust, or droplets • Ingestion. Common exposure scenarios • Manipulation of vials • Opening ampoules • Expelling air from syringes • Drug administration by all routes • Spiking IV bags and changing IV tubing • Leakage of tubing or IV bags or syringes • Contamination of objects in the environment • Handling body fluids of patients who have received chemotherapy • Cleaning up spills	• Discussion and question-and-answer session with instructor • Review of clinical setting for possible exposure scenarios by walking through and observing administration of chemotherapy Learner will journal about practices observed and identify potential areas for improvement.

Demonstrate safe handling, administration, and disposal of hazardous drugs in accordance with recommended best practices.	Overview of appropriate drug storage, transportation, handling, and disposal procedures
	• NIOSH alert regarding safe handling of hazardous drugs, drug handling, and disposal
	• Review and practice safe handling techniques using PPE, including gloves, gowns, respirator, and eye and face protection
	• Rationale for PPE use
	• Review work practice controls to minimize environmental contamination, such as not spiking at the bedside, working below eye level, using PPE, using closed-system devices if available, using gauze under syringe at injection ports, using Luer-lock connections when possible, safe priming of IV tubing, washing exposed surfaces with detergent and water, and proper disposal technique.
	• Standard precautions, including double gloving and disposable gowns, when handling excreta of patients who have received hazardous drugs in previous 48 hours
	• Use of face protection when splashing is possible
		• Clinical observation with patients receiving chemotherapy
		• Under supervision of instructor, performance of
		  – Return demonstration of appropriate PPE use while administering hazardous drugs
		  – Return demonstration of work practice controls to minimize environmental contamination
		  – Return demonstration of proper disposal technique utilizing hazardous waste receptacles
		  – Instructing patient and family on safe handling practices, including hand-washing, PPE, safety of children and pets, management of linens and contaminated objects
		  – Locating spill kit and reviewing contents
		
		Materials:
		• NIOSH alert
		• Oncology Nursing Society (ONS) *Chemotherapy and Biotherapy Guidelines and Recommendations for Practice*, Appendix 5, Cancer Chemotherapy Administration Competency Record (Polovich et al., 2009, p. 356)

(Continued on next page)

Appendix B. Hazardous Drug Administration Practicum for RNs *(Continued)*

Objectives	Content	Teaching/Learning Strategies
Demonstrate safe handling, administration, and disposal of hazardous drugs in accordance with recommended best practices. *(Cont.)*	• Use of leakproof pads for inpatients or patients at home • Linen handling procedures • Review of spill management procedures according to best practice	• *ONS Chemotherapy and Biotherapy Guidelines and Recommendations for Practice,* Appendix 3, Safe Management of Chemotherapy in the Home (Polovich et al., 2009, pp. 353–354) • Spill kit matching game to identify use of each component In advance of clinical experience, learner will download and review *CDC Workplace Solutions: Personal Protective Equipment for Health Care Workers Who Work With Hazardous Drugs* (www.cdc.gov/niosh/docs/wp-solutions/2009-106/pdfs/2009-106.pdf).
Explain the concept of medical surveillance as a component of a safe handling program.	Definition of medical surveillance • Comprehensive program to minimize workplace exposure • Engineering controls • Work practices • PPE Elements of a medical surveillance program • Health surveys • Laboratory work • Physical examination • Rationale for follow-ups	• Discussion with preceptor • Visit to occupational health for medical surveillance program enrollment In advance of clinical experience, learner will download and review *Medical Surveillance for Health Care Workers Exposed to Hazardous Drugs* (www.cdc.gov/niosh/docs/wp-solutions/2007-117/pdfs/2007-117.pdf).

Index

The letter *f* after a page number indicates that relevant content appears in a figure; the letter *t*, in a table.

A

acute symptoms, of HD exposure, 10–11, 60–61
administrative controls, 18, 23, 70
adult learning, strategies for, 70–71
adverse effects, of HD exposure, 4–11, 5*t*–10*t*
aerosol HD administration, 43. *See also* inhalation exposure
air changes per hour (ACPH), 21
airflow, in BSCs, 19, 31
air quality measurement, 18, 21
alemtuzumab, 32
American Hospital Formulary Service (AHFS), 4*t*
American Society for Testing and Materials (ASTM), 25
American Society of Health-System Pharmacists (ASHP), 3, 36
ampoules, HDs supplied in, 32–33
ante area, in PEC, 19*f*, 21
arsenic trioxide, 32, 48*f*, 51*f*, 52
aseptic technique, 32. *See also* sterile preparations, compounding of
Association for Linen Management, 50

B

barriers, to safe handling practices, 71–72
B cabinets, 19. *See also* biologic safety cabinets
biologic effects, of HD exposure, 5, 6*t*–10*t*
biologic monitoring, for medical surveillance, 11–12, 60, 63–64
biologic safety cabinets (BSCs), 12, 18–20, 61, 68
  decontamination of, 28–31, 29*t*
  drug compounding in, 28–31
  limitations of, 31
  spill cleanup within, 56. *See also* spill management
blood-brain barrier (BBB), 43
body fluids, 47–49, 48*t*, 48*f*, 54*t*
breast milk, HDs secreted in, 48, 48*f*
broken glass, 56
buffer area, in PEC, 19*f*, 21

C

calcium hypochlorite, 55
cancer occurrence, in HD-exposed HCWs, 11
carboplatin, 13
carcinogenicity, 3, 51*f*, 68
carmustine, 15*t*, 25, 48*t*
carpeting, HD spills on, 56

cerebrospinal fluid (CSF), 43
characteristic waste, 52
checklist, for safe handling practices, 83
Chemoplus™ Prep Mat, 31
chlorambucil, 52
chromosomal aberrations, from HD exposure, 5
cisplatin, 12–13, 15*t*–16*t*, 48*t*, 48*f*
cleaning, of PECs, 20, 28–30, 29*t*
closed-system drug transfer devices (CSTDs), 21–23, 33, 36–37, 68
coliseum technique, of HD administration, 47
compliance, with safe handling practices, 66–67, 71
compounded sterile preparations (CSPs), 27. *See also* compounding
compounding
  of nonsterile preparations, 34
  of sterile preparations, 18–19, 27–34
compounding aseptic containment isolators (CACIs), 18, 20–21, 28, 30
conjugated estrogens, 3
constitutional symptoms, 61
containers, for hazardous waste, 52–53
continuous infusion, 45
conversational learning, 72
cradle-to-grave tracking, of HDs, 52–53
crushing, of HDs, 37–38
cyclophosphamide, 5, 12–13, 14*t*–17*t*, 21, 25, 48, 48*f*, 51*f*, 52

D

daunorubicin, 52
deactivation, of HDs, 20, 28–30, 29*t*, 55
decontamination, of PECs, 20, 28–30, 29*t*, 35
dermal exposure/absorption, 10–11, 13, 38, 57, 68
detergent solutions, 55
dialysis, 46
diethylstilbestrol, 52
disinfection, of PECs, 20, 28–30, 29*t*, 35
disposal
  of hazardous waste, 30, 35–36, 51*f*, 51–53
  of PPE, 53
DNA damage, from HD exposure, 5
docetaxel, 15*t*, 48*t*
documentation
  of drug-handling history, 64–65
  of spills/accidents, 61
dosage verification, 24
double bagging, of laundry, 50
double flushing, 48–49

double gloving, 24, 26, 31, 34
doxorubicin, 15t, 25, 48t, 48f
drapes, in PECs, 31
drug administration, 35–47, 36f
drug compounding. *See* compounding
drug-handling history, of HCW, 64–65
drug vials
    contamination on, 13, 30
    labeling on, 30, 34–35
dry-spike adapters, 22, 34, 36

E

education, of staff, 66–72
    checklist for, 83
    practicum for, 84–85
    strategies for, 70–71
effusions, 42, 48
emesis, 48. *See also* body fluids
engineering controls, 18–23, 19f
    staff training on, 68, 70
enteral/enterostomy tubes, 37f, 37–38
environmental monitoring, 12–13, 14t–17t
epidural catheters, 44
etoposide, 15t, 25, 48t, 48f, 51f
evidence, for HD exposure, 11–13, 14t–17t
excreta, 48–49, 54t. *See also* body fluids
exemestane, 48f
exposure history, for medical surveillance, 60
exposure, routes of, 10–11, 13, 38, 57, 68–69
eye, HD administration through, 44
eye protection, 27, 68
eyewash stations, 27, 57

F

face shields, 27, 68
fertility impairment, 3, 10, 51f, 58, 68
floor contamination, 19–20, 46
fluorouracil, 13, 14t–17t, 21, 25
follow-up, after accidental exposure, 57, 64
fume hoods, 19, 34

G

ganciclovir, 3
gemcitabine, 48t
genetic damage, from HD exposure, 5, 11
genotoxicity, 3, 51f, 67–68
glass, broken, 56
gloves, 25–26, 26f, 66–68
    changing/discarding of, 12, 24–25, 30–32
    contamination on/under, 13, 31
    testing of, 25
    use in PECs, 31–32
goggles, 27
goserelin, 48f
gowns, 26–27, 31, 34, 66–68, 71

H

hands, as common exposure site, 13
hazardous drugs (HDs), definition of, 3–4, 4t, 51, 51f
Hazardous Material Response Team, for HD spills, 54
hazardous waste, 30, 35–36, 51f, 51–53
health effects, of HD exposure, 5–11, 6t–10t, 68
hemodialysis, 46
HEPA (high-efficiency particulate air) filters, 18–19, 56
hierarchy of controls, 18f, 18–27
high-fidelity simulators, 72
history
    of exposure, for medical surveillance, 60–61, 62f–63f
    of HD handling, 64–65
home setting
    double flushing in, 49
    HD administration in, 69–70
    HD spills in, 56
    linen care in, 50
hyperthermic IP chemotherapy, 47

I

ifosfamide, 12–13, 14t–17t, 21
imatinib, 48, 48t, 48f
implanted reservoirs, 44
implanted time-release delivery, 43
incidence reports, for spills, 56
incontinence, 49, 49f. *See also* body fluids
industrial hygiene, 18
Infusaid™ Pump, 44–45
ingestion exposure, 57, 68
inhalation exposure, 13, 42, 57, 68
injection, HD administration by, 36–37
interferon alpha, 3, 48t
International Agency for Research on Cancer (IARC), 3, 4t
International Organization for Standardization (ISO), 18, 19f, 21
interventional settings, for HD administration, 46–47
intra-arterial delivery, 45
intracavitary HD administration, 38
intracerebral HD administration, 44
intramuscular injections, 37
intraocular HD administration, 44
intraoperative HD administration, 47, 69
intraperitoneal (IP) delivery, 41–42, 47, 69
intrapleural HD administration, 42
intraspinal HD administration, 43–44
intrathecal HD administration, 43–44
intravenous infusions, 36
intravenous injections, 36–37
intraventricular HD administration, 43
intravesicular HD administration, 41, 69
isolators, 20
isopropyl alcohol
    for disinfection, 28, 29t, 30
    and glove integrity, 26
IV bag adapters, 22, 34, 36

L

labels/labeling
   damaged from disinfectants, 30
   for drug-handling history tracking, 65
   of hazardous waste, 52–53
   of HDs, 34–35
laboratory studies, for medical surveillance,
      60–63, 63*f*, 64
latex gloves, 26
latex sensitivity, 26
laundry, 49*f*, 49–50
learning styles, in adult learners, 71
linen handling, 49*f*, 49–50
listed wastes, 52
locking connectors, 22, 32, 34, 36
lomustine, 48*f*
Luer connectors, 22, 32, 34, 36
lumbar puncture, 43–44

M

malignant pleural effusions (MPEs), 42
material safety data sheets (MSDSs), 4*t*, 57
medical history, 60–61, 62*f*–63*f*
medical surveillance, 23, 57–59, 69
   elements of, 59*f*, 59–64, 62*f*–63*f*
megestrol acetate, 48*f*
melphalan, 51*f*, 52
mercaptopurine, 48*f*
methotrexate, 5, 14*t*, 17*t*, 48, 48*t*, 48*f*
MiniMed™ Programmable Implantable
      Infusion System, 44
mitomycin, 48*f*, 51*f*, 52
mitoxantrone, 48*t*, 48*f*

N

nasogastric/nasoenteric tubes, 37*f*, 37–38
National Institute for Occupational Safety
      and Health (NIOSH), 4, 4*t*, 23
   on drug compounding, 27–28
   on unspiking, 36
National Toxicology Program, 4*t*
nebulized therapy, 43. *See also* inhalation
      exposure
needle-safe/needle-free connections, 22, 32,
      36
negative pressure technique, 32–33
neutralizers, 28–30, 29*t*
nitrile gloves, 26
noncompliance, with safe handling practices,
      66–67, 71
nonmalignant conditions, treated with HDs,
      35*f*
nonsterile preparations, compounding of, 34
nontraditional settings, for HD delivery, 45–47

O

Occupational Safety and Health
      Administration (OSHA), 3, 18, 27, 66
Ommaya reservoirs, 44
ONS Chemotherapy and Biotherapy Course,
      70

open abdomen technique, of HD administra-
      tion, 47
operative settings, for HD administration,
      46–47, 69
oral HDs, 34, 37–38, 39*t*–40*t*
organ toxicity, 3, 51*f*

P

package inserts, 4*t*, 57
paclitaxel, 25, 51*f*
pass-throughs, in PECs, 28
P codes, 52
percutaneous HD administration, 45
peritoneum, 41
permeation testing, for gloves/gowns, 25–26
personal protective equipment (PPE), 10,
      12–13, 18, 25–27, 26*f*, 66–67. *See also*
      gloves; gowns; respirators
   disposal of, 53
   HCW's history of use, 61
   in PECs, 31–32
   for spill cleanup, 55–56
   staff education on, 66–68
pheresis, 46
physical examination, for medical surveil-
      lance, 60–61
platinum-containing HDs, 12–13, 15*t*–16*t*. *See
      also specific agents*
policies/procedures. *See* administrative con-
      trols
polifeprosan 20 with carmustine implant,
      43
polyethylene gowns, 26, 71
polymer wafers, 43
polypropylene gowns, 26
powder-free gloves, 25
practicum, for safe handling training, 84–85
primary engineering control (PEC), 13,
      18–19, 19*f*, 27
   cleaning/disinfecting of, 28–30, 29*t*
   drug compounding in, 28
   PPE in, 31–32
   work practices in, 28–31, 29*t*
priming IV lines, 33–34, 54*t*
professional groups, education/training by,
      70
provider cards, 70

R

radiation exposure, 11
RCRA-empty designation, for waste contain-
      ers, 52–53
reconstitution, of HDs, 32, 54*t*
record keeping
   of drug-handling history, 64–65
   of spills/accidents, 61
reproductive history, for medical surveil-
      lance, 61, 68
reproductive toxicity, 3, 10, 51*f*, 58, 61
respirators, 27, 43, 45, 55, 68
role modeling, of safe handling practices, 72
routes of exposure, 10–11, 13, 38, 42–43, 57,
      68–69

S

sanitizing, 29t. *See also* disinfection, of PECs
simulated practice, 72
skin exposure, to HDs, 10–11, 13, 38, 57, 68
sodium hypochlorite (bleach) solution,
    28–30, 29t, 55–56
sodium thiosulfate solution, 29t, 55
spiking IV bags, 33–34, 36, 54t
spill kits, 54, 56
spill management, 53–57, 54t, 55f
staff education/training, 66–72
    checklist for, 83
    practicum for, 84–85
    strategies for, 70–71
sterile preparations, compounding of,
    18–19, 27–34
streptozocin, 48f, 52
subcutaneous injections, 37
sunitinib, 48
surface contamination, 12–13, 14t–17t, 21
surface decontamination, 20, 28–30, 29t, 35
Surface Safe® decontaminant, viii, 30, 55–56
surface wipe sampling, 12–13, 14t–17t
surgical masks, 27
sweat, 48. *See also* body fluids
symptoms
    acute, 10–11, 60–61
    constitutional, 61
SynchroMed® drug delivery system, 44

T

tacrolimus, 32, 48f
temsirolimus, 48t
Tenckhoff catheters, 42
teniposide, 48t
teratogenicity, 3, 51f
thalidomide, 3
thiotepa, 25
topical HDs, 38
trace contamination, 52
tracking, of HDs, 52–53
training, of staff, 66–72
    checklist for, 83
    practicum for, 84–85

strategies for, 70–71
transfer chambers, in PECs, 28
tretinoin, 48f

U

U codes, 52
unit-dose packaging, 34, 37
United States Pharmacopeia (USP), 18, 19f,
    20–21, 28, 30
unspiking HD bags, 36, 54t
urinary mutagenicity, from HD exposure, 5
urine, HD detection in, 11–12. *See also* body
    fluids

V

Vacutainer® system, 49
valrubicin, 51f
variance reports, for spills, 56
ventilated cabinets, 18–19
vials. *See* drug vials
vincristine, 48t, 48f
vinorelbine, 48t
vinyl gowns, 26, 71
virtual patients, 72

W

wafers, implantable, 43
Washburn setup, for tube administration, 38,
    41, 41f, 42
waste containers, 52–53
waste disposal, 30, 35–36, 51f, 51–53
waste outlets, in PECs, 30, 35
wipes, 30
work history, for medical surveillance, 61
work practice controls, 24–25
    in PECs, 28–31, 29t
    staff training on, 68–70

Z

zidovudine, 48f